DIABETIC COOKBOOK FOR BEGINNERS

THE MUST-HAVE GUIDE ON HOW TO MANAGE TYPE 1-2 DIABETES THROUGH THE FOOD.

A 30-DAY MEAL PLAN WITH HEALTHY, EASY, AND TASTY RECIPES FOR THE NEWLY DIAGNOSED INCLUDED.

Erica Diason

TABLE OF CONTENTS

CHAPTER 16. DESSERTS AND SNACKS RECIPES 159

INTRODUCTION

The risk of contracting chronic diseases is minimized by healthy eating habits. This can have an impact on your energy levels and how you feel on a daily basis.

To keep you alive, your body needs oxygen. Choosing whole, healthy foods will give the body the nutrients it requires to perform at its best much of the time. You can find that they affect your energy levels as well as your health if you consume a lot of refined foods high in sugar and fat. In addition, you can lose out on the required nutrients if you have an irregular meal schedule and skip meals daily, leaving you feeling exhausted.

One research showed that it was much more likely for students who missed breakfast or had an erratic eating routine involving skipping meals daily to feel exhaustion. It's also crucial that during the day, you eat enough food to sustain yourself. The lack of both calories and vital nutrients, such as iron, will result in drastic dietary limitations, which will adversely affect the energy levels. A diet based on whole grains helps your health and your energy balance with nutritious foods. In comparison, the energy levels will be adversely influenced by a diet rich in refined foods.

A sweet, sugar-filled snack can be easy to reach for when you feel sleepy. However, while sugar will provide you with a short-term energy boost, it will easily wear off. This is because, often referred to as a blood sugar surge, high-sugar foods cause blood sugar to increase rapidly. This results in massive quantities of insulin being released by the body to get your blood sugar back down. This rise and fall in blood sugar are thought to be what triggers a surge of energy followed by a slump. One research, for example, found that adults consuming a sugar-filled breakfast cereal classified themselves as more exhausted than those consuming a more complicated carbohydrate breakfast cereal. Complex carbohydrates are absorbed into the bloodstream more slowly.

Your chances of obesity, diabetes, and heart disease may also be raised by consuming high quantities of added sugar, so reducing added sugar in your diet is not only beneficial for your energy levels but also for your health. Try eliminating foods rich in added sugar to keep the energy levels more stable and decrease fatigue.

By eating whole and fiber-rich ingredients, such as whole grains, vegetables, and legumes, you will increase the consistency of your diet. A short-term energy gain followed by a slump may be provided by consuming foods rich in sugar. Minimize the diet to prevent this and rely more on choosing whole foods. Your first concern of high blood sugar is probably when you hear the term "diabetes." An often-underestimated part of your well-being is blood sugar. It could turn into diabetes when it's out of whack for a long period of time. The capacity of your body to generate or use insulin, a hormone that helps your body to convert glucose (sugar) into energy, is impaired by diabetes. Here are the signs your body can experience as diabetes takes place.

When caught early, diabetes can be easily controlled. However, it can lead to possible risks that include heart failure, stroke, kidney injury, and nerve damage when left untreated.

Your body would usually break down the carbohydrates from your diet after you consume or drink and use them as energy in your cells. Your pancreas needs to generate a hormone called insulin to do this. Insulin is what makes it possible to pull sugar from the blood and transfer it into the cells for consumption or for electricity.

Your pancreas either contains very little insulin or none at all if you have diabetes. It's difficult to use insulin successfully. As the majority of your cells are depleted of much-needed resources, this causes blood glucose levels to increase. This can lead to a wide spectrum of complications involving virtually any single system of the body.

The effects of diabetes on your body depend substantially on the type of diabetes you suffer from. Two key forms of diabetes exist, type 1 and type 2.

A deficiency of the immune system is type 1, also called juvenile diabetes or insulin-dependent diabetes. In the pancreas, your own immune system destroys the insulin-producing cells, killing the capacity of the body to make insulin. Type 1 diabetes necessitates the use of insulin. As an infant or young adult, most persons are diagnosed.

Type 2 is insulin resistance-related. It used to exist in older populations, but now type 2 diabetes is diagnosed in increasingly younger populations. This is a product of poor health, nutritional, and fitness patterns. Your pancreas ceases using insulin properly in type 2 diabetes. This creates complications with being able to take sugar out of the blood and put it for energy in the cells. Finally, this will add to the need for insulin treatment.

Earlier levels, such as pre-diabetes, can be controlled successfully with food, exercise, and diligent blood sugar control. The complete progression of type 2 diabetes will also be avoided by this. It is possible to monitor diabetes. It may also go into remission in some cases if proper lifestyle changes are made.

High blood sugar, which occurs during breastfeeding, is gestational diabetes. You can manage gestational diabetes much of the time by diet and exercise. Usually, it even operates until the infant is born. During pregnancy, gestational diabetes will increase the risk of complications. It will also raise the likelihood that both mothers and children may experience type 2 diabetes later in life.

We will explain in depth about diabetes, forms of diabetes, causes of diabetes, signs of diabetes, management of diabetes, means and methods of avoiding and managing diabetes, how healthy diet and healthy lifestyle lead to reducing and managing the adverse consequences of diabetes and finally the prescribed foods to be consumed and banned foods to be avoided during diabetes. This book includes several recipes for a healthy lifestyle that a diabetic person can select from.

CHAPTER 1. UNDERSTANDING THE DIABETES

According to the CDC, there are more than 30 million individuals in America that have diabetes; and 1 in 4 of these people don't know they have this condition. The cause of diabetes is linked with the pancreases, which fails to produce or use insulin properly. Insulin hormone is secreted into the bloodstream by the pancreatic gland to deliver it into the cells. Once the cells take in the sugar, it is then converted into energy and use immediately or store for later use.

1. The Link Between Obesity and Type 2 Diabetes

Although the exact cause of type 2 diabetes is still not fully understood, being obese and overweight is believed to account for 80% of the risk of developing diabetes. So, if you have excess weight around your tummy, you are at greater risk of developing type 2 diabetes. In obese people, the abdominal fat cells have more nutrients than average, and then this stress in the cell makes them release pro-inflammatory chemicals. These chemicals disrupt the function of the insulin hormone and/or make the body less sensitive to insulin. It is called insulin resistance, which is the major cause of type 2 diabetes. Therefore, having excess abdominal fat or a large waistline leads to a high risk of diabetes.

2. Types of Diabetes, Symptoms, and Treatment

There are two main types of diabetes—type 1 diabetes and type 2 diabetes. How can you discover if you have diabetes and which one? The differences between them are their causes.

Type 1 Diabetes

It's an autoimmune disease that causes insulin to destroy the beta cells of the pancreases. It is caused by a fault in the immune response of the body, triggered by a virus, which mistakenly led the body to target and destroy beta cells of the pancreases, which are responsible for producing insulin. Hence, the loss of these cells prevents the body from producing enough insulin to control the blood sugar levels, and the symptoms of diabetes begin to appear.

Signs of type 1 diabetes: This type of diabetes tends to develop more in over 35 years old adults than in children. The signs of type 1 diabetes include increased thirst, dry mouth, peeing more often, itchy skin, weight loss, tiredness during the day, and genital itchiness. If your body shows any of these signs, then there are chances that you have developed diabetes. Consult a doctor immediately, and he may do urine and blood test to confirm if you have actually developed diabetes.

Treatment of type 1 diabetes: As the killing of beta cells reduces insulin in the body, it is the treatment for this condition—insulin treatment. Individuals suffering from type 1 diabetes treat this condition by injecting insulin into the body with an insulin pen and insulin pump. These insulin doses are also balanced with dietary intake, physical activities, and regular monitoring of blood glucose levels that will help you control your diabetes. As mentioned before, exercise and eating healthy meals are important for minimizing the harmful effects of diabetes like retinopathy, kidney diseases, heart diseases, and stroke, etc. However, delivering insulin in the body, proper dietary intake, along exercise only help to maintain a good blood glucose level, not elevating or reversing type 1 diabetes.

Type 2 Diabetes

High blood glucose level results in type 2 diabetes. Under this condition, the body becomes insulin resistant, which is the body becoming ineffective to use insulin hormone and/or it becomes unable to produce insulin. Insulin hormone is needed for cells to take in glucose (simple sugar) from the blood and then convert it into energy. In type 2 diabetes, the body is unable to metabolize simple sugar or glucose, which leads to high blood glucose levels over time that may damage organs of the body. From this, food for individuals suffering from this type of diabetes becomes a sort of poison. But these people can stay well by lowering their blood sugar by avoiding foods that are high in sugar and using some medications.

Signs of type 2 diabetes: The signs of type 2 diabetes are increased urination, increased thirst, and hunger, unintended loss of muscle mass, extreme tiredness, blurred vision, slow healing of sores, frequent infections, and darkened skin under mock and armpits. These symptoms are similar to type 1 diabetes; however, these signs develop more slowly in type 2 diabetes-like over the months and years, and hence, it becomes harder to identify these signs of diabetes.

Risks of type 2 diabetes: There are a number of factors that increase the risk of developing type 2 diabetes, including overweight, consuming unhealthy foods, less physical activity, raised blood pressure, high cholesterol level, smoking, etc. Moreover, environmental factors, family history, age of over 45 years, and belonging to certain races like Asian-American, black, American Indian, and Hispanic also influenced the likelihood of developing diabetes.

Treatment of type 2 diabetes: Irrespective to type 1 diabetes, type 2 diabetes can be prevented if detected and treated at an early stage. The common treatment for type 2 diabetes includes consuming a low carb, high fiber, and low glycemic index diet along with appropriate and regular physical activities. Some medicines may also be prescribed to diabetic patients, like metformin that is the most common drug for type 2 diabetes patients and helps the body to respond better to insulin.

Gestational Diabetes

Hyperglycemia with blood glucose levels over average but below those diabetes levels is diagnosed with gestational diabetes. Gestational diabetes is identified via prenatal tests rather than by signs recorded—high blood sugar, which also occurs during gestation. Hormones produced by the placenta are Insulin-blocking, which is the main cause of this type of diabetes. You can manage gestational diabetes much of the time by food and exercise. Usually, it gets resolved after delivery. During pregnancy, gestational diabetes will raise the risk of complications. It will also increase the likelihood that both mothers and infants may experience type 2 diabetes later in life. This form of diabetes is caused by the placenta's production of insulin-blocking hormones.

CHAPTER 2. DIABETES AND OBESITY

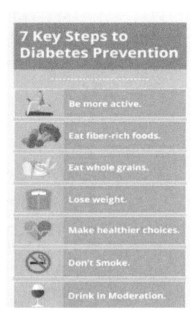

Diabetes is a stubborn condition that arises from two reasons when the pancreas cannot produce Insulin enough for body needs or whenever the Insulin it provides may not be utilized properly by the body. Insulin is a blood sugar-regulating hormone. Hyperglycemia, or high blood sugar, is a typical result of uncontrolled diabetes, causing significant harm to the body's structures, especially blood vessels and nerves over time. Diabetes mellitus is a category of illnesses that influence how the body uses glucose. Glucose is essential to your well-being. The cells that make up the muscles and tissues require a significant supply of glucose. It's the brain's primary power supply, too. The primary issue of diabetes varies based on the type of diabetes. And this can result in excessive sugar in the blood, no matter what kind of diabetes a person has. If there is too much sugar, it can lead to grave health issues. The insulin hormone transfers the sugar into the cells from the blood.

High levels of blood sugar may cause harm to your kidneys, eyes, organs, and nerves.

To understand what is the main reason for diabetes, you should know what the normal route of glucose consumption in the body is.

3. How Glucose and Insulin Work Together

- The pancreas is an organ situated behind and below the stomach that produces Insulin. It is a hormone that regulates the level of sugar in the blood. Here is a step-by-step production in the bloodstream; insulin comes from the pancreases.

- Then Insulin helps the sugar to go into the body cells.

- Insulin reduces the level of sugar in the blood.

- Now that the level of sugar drops in blood, it also causes the pancreas to secret less amount of Insulin.

- As blood sugar level drops in the body, it reduces insulin secretion from the pancreas.

4. The Causes of Diabetes

Causes of Type 1 Diabetes

Type 1 diabetes has an uncertain etiology. It's understood that the immune system targets and eradicates the cells (in the pancreas) that produce Insulin. The immune system usually destroys viruses or infectious bacteria. This leaves little or no insulin for the human body. Sugar keeps building up in the bloodstream instead of being transferred into the cells.

Type 1 diabetes is believed to be triggered by a mixture of hereditary susceptibility and the environment's variables, but it is still uncertain precisely what those variables are. It is not assumed that weight is a variable in type 1 diabetes. Type1 develops as the pancreas' beta cells that produce Insulin are targeted and killed by the body's immune system, the body's ability to combat infection. Scientists assume that type 1 diabetes is triggered by genetic makeup and environmental causes that could induce the condition.

Causes of Prediabetes and Type 2 Diabetes

Your cells can become immune to Insulin's effect in prediabetes, which can happen in type 2 diabetes, and the pancreas is not able to generate sufficient insulin to counteract this resistance. Sugar starts building up in your bloodstream instead of going to your cells, where it's required for fuel. Although genetic and environmental factors are believed to play a role in the development of type 2 diabetes, it is unclear why this occurs. The advancement of type 2 diabetes is closely related to being overweight, although not everybody with type 2 is obese. Several variables, including dietary conditions and genetic makeup, are responsible for the most prevalent type of diabetes.

Here are a few factors:

- **Insulin resistance**

Type 2 diabetes commonly progresses with insulin resistance, a disease in which Insulin is not handled well by the body, liver, and fat cells. As a consequence, to enable glucose to reach cells, the body requires more Insulin. The pancreas initially generates more Insulin to maintain the additional demand. The pancreas can't create enough insulin over time, and blood glucose levels increase.

- **Overweight, physical inactivity, and obesity**

When you are not regularly involved and are obese or overweight, you are much more prone to have type 2 diabetes. Often, excess weight induces insulin resistance, which is prominent in persons with type 2 diabetes. In which the fat stores of the body count a lot. Insulin tolerance, type 2 diabetes, heart, and blood artery dysfunction are attributed to excess belly fat.

- **Genes and family history**

A family history of diabetes in the family makes it more probable that gestational diabetes may occur in a mother, which means that genes play a part. In African Americans, Asians, American Indians, and Latinas, Hispanic, mutations can also justify why the disease happens more frequently.

Any genes can make you more susceptible to advance type 2 diabetes type 1 diabetes.

Genetic makeup can make a person more obese, which in turn leads to having type 2 diabetes.

CHAPTER 3. PRACTICAL SOLUTIONS TO PREVENT/TREAT DIABETES

5. How Can Diabetes Be Prevented and Controlled?

Although medically diabetes has no cure, minor lifestyle changes will go a long way in preventing or controlling the disease. While type 1 diabetes requires regular monitoring by a doctor, type 2 diabetes can be controlled by following a healthy lifestyle.

The idea behind this effort is to identify the factors leading to the pre-diabetes phase, which is just before the onset of diabetes. While a person cannot change the genes leading to diabetes, all of us can put the disease in check when it starts to build up excessive blood sugar levels.

Some common things to do to avoid being affected by diabetes:

Control sugar and carbohydrate intake: One of the basic steps that your doctor will advise you to take is to limit your intake of sugar, carbs, and processed food items. Elevating your sugar intake will lead to extra pressure on the pancreas to produce insulin from which to derive energy for cells by breaking down the sugars in food. This is one of the common ways to trigger type 2 diabetes in young and adults.

Exercise regularly: With everything being handed to us on a platter thanks to the bane of the technologically enabled lifestyle, most of us underutilize our bodies. Lack of physical movement, along with excessive intake of food, has made obesity a household ailment. When a person regularly exercises, the process activates the cells in the body to function even in a condition of low insulin. This allows the insulin to break down the sugar into energy for the cells easily—and, in turn, for the body. A person diagnosed with type 2 diabetes can keep the ailment at bay without taking medication, provided they exercise regularly.

Drink water: Water is one of the main elements of the human body and a great caretaker for people diagnosed with diabetes. Drinking water more frequently rather than relying on other beverages helps you avoid the non-essential carbs and sugar that one can intake by drinking aerated drinks. People who consume soda or aerated drinks as their first choice of beverage are more likely to develop LADA a type 1 diabetes.

Lose weight: Being overweight is one of the precursors to type 2 diabetes. Therefore, a person should be careful to ensure that they are not becoming obese. One of the easiest methods is to check your body mass index regularly. The reading will give you a fair idea of whether you are starting to grow extra fat in your body. Even a small amount of fat gain greatly affects your chances of attracting diabetes. Follow a healthy diet plan and start working out as soon as possible.

Do not smoke: Other than causing life-threatening cancer, smoking wildly affects a diabetic patient. Not just smoking but also second-hand smoke has been shown to have signs of aggravating type 2 diabetes. Get counseling if necessary, but quit smoking. Need we say more?

6. Preventing Pre-diabetes

Prevention is always better than cure. If you can stop yourself from developing diabetes before you actually have it, you will be saving yourself from a lifetime of being a prisoner to your body. It isn't even all that difficult.

Research has proven that if you are pre-diabetic, you can decrease the chances of the onset of type 2 diabetes by losing 7% of your body mass and following a moderate exercise routine. Something as easy as a daily walk around your neighborhood could save your life.

Should you already have type 2 diabetes, this is not a death sentence. You are not a "deadman walking," and by maintaining a healthy weight, engaging in regular exercise, and eating wisely, you can improve your body's acceptance of insulin, thereby decreasing the sugar levels in your blood. You can lock the moody diabetes teenager away and live a healthy and fulfilling life.

7. Diabetes Treatment Options

Treating diabetes is not about getting rid of some boogie in your life. Instead, it is about management. Once diagnosed as diabetic, most people don't get magically diabetic. This means you can't hide in your closet and refuse to deal with the reality and impact of diabetes on your health.

You need to use medical treatment, dietary treatment, and a combination of physical activity and balanced mental health to keep yourself in good health.

8. Medical Treatment

When treating and managing your diabetes, you need to know your blood sugar levels. If you don't know your "sweet spot," you won't be able to regulate your intake of carbohydrates or sucrose and the production of insulin. For type 1 diabetes, this becomes crucial as you may need to take insulin injections to help regulate your blood sugar.

Testing your blood sugar levels isn't like randomly checking your bank balance at the ATM. You need to be organized—your life may depend on it.

When you are diagnosed as a person with diabetes, you need to be prepared and diligent in your testing:

- Always keep your testing equipment with you.
- Use new testing strips and keep them away from heat and sunlight.
- Make testing part of your life and test at the same times each day.
- Schedule maintenance and calibration of your testing machine regularly.
- Keep track of your results in a notebook or app on your phone.
- Manage your testing site effectively and safely.

Knowing your sugar levels are helps you plan your diet and enables you to manage your diabetes with careful nutrition planning.

9. Dietary Treatment

Medical Nutrition Therapy (MNT) is when your healthcare practitioner advises you about which foods to avoid, which to bulk on, and times and quantities of your meals. This helps your body work in sync with your unique diabetes diagnosis. No two diabetics are identical, and while you can maybe sneak a candy bar once in a while, your neighbor may have fits if they have even one sniff of chocolate.

In numerous tests and research studies, the DASH diet, the Mediterranean diet, and vegetarian or plant-based foods have been found to be the most beneficial to those managing their diabetes. After all, you are what you eat.

A structured meal plan can really help you get those blood sugar numbers under control. By following a specially crafted MNT, you can cut down on the blood glucose levels in your body, reducing your blood sugar levels, and maintaining optimal health. This puts you in control of your diabetes with every spoonful you eat.

10. Physical Activity and Mental Health

Get up and move. Not only will this help you produce endorphins that will help you feel better, but it will also reduce your blood glucose levels. Even if you don't necessarily lose weight with your physical activities, it is still a win for anyone living with diabetes.

Try to get at least two and a half hours of physical activity throughout a week. Be careful to spread that feel-good movement over a couple of days. Never do more than two consecutive days of exercise. Not only will this help prevent injuries, but it will also help you form healthy physical activity habits.

Living with diabetes can be overwhelming, and you need to cultivate a strong mental approach. Type 2 diabetes is particularly rough on your emotions, and you may suffer from mood swings and feel stressed. Engage in self-care, and you will be able to remain mentally and emotionally fit and on top of your game.

If you are going to let sugar become your boss, then your health will suffer. Diabetes management is important to preserve your health and well-being. Stay positive and live responsibly. There is no need to become overwhelmed or depressed (though you may feel like this at times). When in doubt, reach out. There are amazing online support groups. And in many urban centers, there are also diabetes clinics where you can get access to resources and helpful advice from medical professionals.

Diabetes is absolutely treatable, and by following a controlled diet, working with your healthcare practitioners, and maintaining a healthy weight and exercise program (and, if necessary, taking medication), you can beat diabetes.

CHAPTER 4. A HEALTHY MEAL CAN HELP EASE THE EFFECTS OF DIABETES

What you eat matters most when you have diabetes. The good news is that nothing isn't permitted, and even the items which you consider as "bad" for you could be taken in tiny amounts as occasional treats. Still, it's better to stick to the best food options to easily manage your diabetes.

11. Starches

What to eat—The best options are to eat whole grains like millet, oatmeal, quinoa, barley, brown rice, amaranth and high fiber cereals, flours such as coconut flour, almond flour, hazelnut flours, and no or very little added sugar.

What to avoid—Avoid processed grains like white flour, baked goods made with white flour like white bread, white rice, white pasta, crackers, pretzels, cereals with lots of sugar, white flour tortilla, etc.

12. Vegetables

What to eat—You need to eat vegetables that have fewer carbs and lots of fibers, and this includes all fresh and/or frozen vegetables, especially leafy greens. You can eat them raw and have them as roasted, grilled, or steamed. You can also use canned vegetables in your meal but make sure they are unsalted or have low sodium.

What to avoid—Worst choices of vegetables include canned veggies with high sodium, vegetables cooked with lots of high-fat cheeses, butter or sauce, and high sodium pickles.

13. Fruits

What to eat—Eat fruits that are low in fat and sodium and high in fiber, minerals, and vitamins like berries, pears, apples, oranges, etc. But fruits tend to have more carbohydrates than vegetables. The best choices for fruits are fresh fruits, frozen fruits, or canned fruits without any sugar. Similarly, you can eat low-sugar or sugar-free jam and apple sauce.

What to avoid—Avoid eating fruits that have a high glycemic index, canned fruits that are packed in heavy sugar syrup, sweetened applesauce, and regular jelly, jam, and preserves. Avoid taking sweetened fruit punches, drinks, juices, and alcoholic drinks.

14. Proteins

What to eat—Include plant-based proteins in your meals like chickpeas, beans, nuts, and seeds. You can also consume grass-fed beef, pastured chicken, pork and lamb, wild-caught fish in moderate amounts. You can get protein from vegan meat options like tofu and seitan. Add pastured eggs and low-fat cheeses to your food to meet your protein requirements.

What to avoid—Avoid fried and higher fat meat cuts, regular cheeses, poultry with skin, deep-fried tofu, and fish and beans prepared using lard.

15. Dairy

What to eat—Use low-fat dairy but in small portions, and this includes skim or reduced-fat milk, low-fat yogurt, low-fat cheeses, and non-fat sour cream.

What to avoid—Don't use whole milk, regular milk, sweetened yogurt, cheeses, sour cream, half-and-half, and ice creams.

16. Fats, Oils, and Sweets

What to eat—Use natural sources of fats like vegetables, like eating nuts, seeds, olives, avocado, reduced-fat dips and dressing, and plant-based oils like olive oil, canola oil, grapeseed oil, and low-fat butter. You can also eat high-fat fishes like tuna, salmon, and mackerel as these foods are rich in omega-3 fatty acids. For sweetness, use dried fruits or sugar substitutes like coconut sugar, erythritol, swerve, Stevia, etc.

What to avoid—Avoid every food that has trans-fat as it is bad for heart health, even if the nutritional label says the food contains 0 g. trans-fat. Also, avoid big portions of saturated fats like coconut oil, palm oil, or animal products. Don't eat fries, potato chips, most fast foods, and pre-made meals.

17. Drinks

What to eat—The best options for drinks include lots of water, unflavored water, unsweetened tea and black coffee, coffee with low-fat milk, flavored sparkling water, non-fruity drinks, fresh and unsweetened fruit juices, and a small number of wines. Read the labels of the drink to know what is being served to you.

What to avoid—Avoid drinking regular sodas, fruity mixed drinks, wines, sweetened tea, sweetened coffee with high-fat milk and cream, flavored drinks, chocolate drinks, sodas, energy drinks, and sweeteners such a table sugar, maple syrup, agave nectar, etc.

CHAPTER 5. MEAL PLANNING AND YOUR LIFESTYLE

A meal plan tells you what, when, and how much to eat to get the nutrients you need while staying within your target blood sugar range. A healthy meal plan would consider your objectives, preferences, and lifestyle, as well as any medications you're taking.

To prevent high or low blood sugar levels, prepare for normal, well-balanced meals. It will help if you eat about the same amount of carbs at each meal.

Carbohydrates, fat, and fiber all have various effects on blood sugar levels. Carbohydrates can increase blood sugar levels more quickly and significantly than protein or fat. Since carbs with fiber, such as sweet potatoes, can help you control your blood sugar, they won't increase your blood sugar as quickly as carbs with little or no fiber, such as soda.

18. Carb Counting

Taking note of how many carbohydrates you consume and setting a limit for each meal will help you stay within your target blood sugar range. Consult your doctor or a dietitian to determine how many carbs you can consume each day and at each meal, and then use this list of popular carb-containing foods and serving sizes as a guide. See Carb Counting for more detail.

Using the glycemic index external symbol is another way to keep track of your carb intake (GI). Carbohydrates in food are ranked from 0 to 100 on the GI scale based on how much they affect blood sugar. Low-GI foods are digested and consumed more slowly by your body, allowing you to feel fuller for longer. They have no consequences on blood sugar levels. Foods with a high GI are digested and consumed faster. They have a greater effect on your blood sugar and cause you to become hungry more quickly. Here are some examples:

Bread (white and wheat), mashed potatoes, watermelon, and fruit juice have a high GI.

Beans, brown rice, tomatoes, yogurt, apples, and milk are all low GI foods.

19. Shopping List

What to Have on a Diabetic Diet

Vegetables:

Fresh vegetables never cause harm to anyone. So, adding a meal full of vegetables is the best shot for all diabetic patients. But not all vegetables contain the same amount of macronutrient. Some vegetables contain a high amount of carbohydrates, so those are not suitable for a diabetic diet. We need to use vegetables which contain a low amount of carbohydrates.

- Cauliflower
- Spinach
- Tomatoes
- Broccoli
- Lemons
- Artichoke
- Garlic
- Asparagus
- Spring onions
- Onions
- Ginger etc.

Meat:

Meat is not on the red list for the diabetic diet. It is fine to have some meat every now and then for diabetic patients. However, certain meat types are better than others. For instance, red meat is not a preferable option for such patients. They should consume white meat more often, whether it's seafood or poultry. Healthy options in meat are:

- All fish, i.e., salmon, halibut, trout, cod, sardine, etc.
- Scallops
- Mussels
- Shrimp
- Oysters, etc.

Fruits:

Not all fruits are good for diabetes. To know if the fruit is suitable for this diet, it is important to note its sugar content. Some fruits contain a high amount of sugars in the form of sucrose and fructose, and those should be readily avoided. Here is the list of popularly used fruits that can be taken on the diabetic diet:

- Peaches
- Nectarines
- Avocados
- Apples
- Berries
- Grapefruit
- Kiwi Fruit
- Bananas
- Cherries
- Grapes
- Orange
- Pears
- Plums
- Strawberries

Nuts and Seeds:

Nuts and seeds are perhaps the most enriched edibles, and they contain such a mix of macronutrients that can never harm anyone. So diabetic patients can take the nuts and seeds in their diet without any fear of glucose spikes.

- Pistachios
- Sunflower seeds
- Walnuts
- Peanuts
- Pecans
- Pumpkin seeds
- Almonds
- Sesame seeds, etc.

Grains:

Diabetic patients should also be selective while choosing the right grains for their diet. The idea is to keep the amount of starch as minimum as possible. That is why you won't any see any white rice in the list rather, it is replaced with more fibrous brown rice.

- Quinoa
- Oats
- Multigrain
- Whole grains
- Brown rice
- Millet
- Barley
- Sorghum
- Tapioca

Fats:

Fat intake is the most debated topic as far as the diabetic diet is concerned. As there are diets like ketogenic, which are loaded with fats and still proved effective for diabetic patients. The key is the absence of carbohydrates. In any other situation, fats are as harmful to people with diabetes as any average person. Switching to unsaturated fats is a better option.

1. Sesame oil
2. Olive oil
3. Canola oil
4. Grapeseed oil
5. Other vegetable oils
6. Fats extracted from plant sources.

Dairy:

Any dairy product which directly or indirectly causes a glucose rise in the blood should not be taken on this diet. Other than those, all products are good to use. These items include:

- Skimmed milk
- Low-fat cheese
- Eggs
- Yogurt
- Trans-fat-free margarine or butter

Sugar Alternatives:

Since ordinary sugars or sweeteners are strictly forbidden on a diabetic diet. There are artificial varieties that can add sweetness without raising the level of carbohydrates in the meal. These substitutes are:

- Stevia
- Xylitol
- Natvia
- Swerve
- Monk fruit

- Erythritol

Make sure to substitute them with extra care. The sweetness of each sweetener is entirely different from the table sugar, so add each in accordance with the intensity of their flavor. Stevia is the sweetest of them, and it should be used with more care. In place of 1 cup of sugar, a tsp. of Stevia is enough. All other sweeteners are more or less similar to sugar in their intensity of sweetness.

20.   Healthy Living and Healthy Eating Habits

To obtain optimal health benefits, it is necessary to use the right combination of numerous nutrients. Generally, a healthy diet includes the following classes of foods:

- Starchy foods such as potatoes, bread, pasta, and rice in smaller portions.
- Big portions of vegetables and fruits.
- Little amounts of dairy and milk foods.
- Protein foods include meat, fish, eggs.
- Protein (non-dairy), including beans, nuts, pulses, and tofu.
- The fifth food segment that you consume is fatty and sugary goods. Sugary and Fatty things can, though, make up just a limited portion of what you consume.
- Must eat salmon, sardines, and pilchards.
- Must eat dark green vegetables like broccoli and kale.
- Foods enriched in calcium, such as fruit juices and soya goods.
- Vitamin D allows the body to digest calcium, so try to go outdoors to receive vitamin D from the sun, have enough vitamin D-containing items, such as fortified cereal, fatty fish in the diet.
- It's necessary, substitute saturated fat with polyunsaturated fat.
- Consume at least five vegetable and fruit portions a day.
- Consume a minimum of two portions of fish each week (ideally fatty fish).
- Start consuming entire grains and nuts daily.
- Keep the sum of salt to very little, like 6 g a day.
- Restricted the consumption of alcohol.

Limit or Avoid the Following in Diet

- Commercially manufactured or processed meats, or readymade foods that are high in trans fatty acids and salt.

- Refined grains, such as dried cereals or white bread.

- Sweetened sugary beverages.

- High-calorie yet nutritionally weak foods, such as cookies, desserts, and crisps.

A Well-Balanced Diet Includes All the Following

- You need the stamina to be productive during the day.

- Nutrients you need to develop and restore help you remain balanced and powerful and help avoid diet-related diseases, such as diabetes and certain cancers.

- You may also help sustain a healthier weight by staying busy and consuming a healthy, nutritious diet.

- Deficiencies of some vital nutrients, such as vitamins C, A, B, and E, and selenium, zinc, and iron, can impair the immune system's parts.

- You will reduce the chances of developing type 2 diabetes and better heart health and will make your teeth & bones by keeping a healthier weight and consuming a nutritious diet low in saturated fat and rich in fiber that is found in whole grains.

- Eating a balanced diet in the proper amounts, coupled with exercise, will also help you lose weight, lower cholesterol and blood pressure levels, and reduce the chances of type 2 diabetes.

Mg/DL	Fasting	After Eating	2-3 hours After Eating
Normal	80-100	170-200	120-140
Impaired Glucose	101-125	190-230	140-160
Diabetic	126 +	220-300	200 +

21. Tips to Control Diabetes

- *Eat less salt:* Salt can increase your chances of having high blood pressure, which leads to increased chances of heart disease and stroke.

- *Replace sugar:* Replace sugar with zero-calorie sweeteners. Cutting out sugar gives you much more control over your blood sugar levels.

- *Cut out alcohol:* Alcohol tends to be high in calories, and if drunk on an empty stomach with insulin medication, it can cause drastic drops in blood sugar.

- *Be physically active:* it lowers your risk of cardiovascular issues and increases your body's natural glucose burn rate.

- *Avoid saturated fats:* Saturated fats like butter and pastries can lead to high cholesterol and blood circulation issues.

- *Use canola or olive oil:* If you need to use oil in your cooking, use canola or olive oil. Both are high in beneficial fatty acids and monounsaturated fat.

- *Drink water:* Water is by far the healthiest drink you can have. Drinking water helps to regulate blood sugar and insulin levels.

- *Make sure you get enough vitamin D:* Vitamin D is a crucial vitamin for controlling blood sugar levels. Eat food high in this vitamin or ask your doctor about supplements.

- *Avoid processed food:* Processed foods tend to be high in vegetable oils, salt, refined grains, or other unhealthy additives.

- *Drink coffee and tea:* Not only are coffee and tea great hunger suppressants for dieters, but they contain important antioxidants that help with protecting cells.

CHAPTER 6. DIETARY REQUIREMENTS OF DIABETICS

When treating diabetes, nutrition is a key component that should be deliberated. A balanced meal plan will help you control your blood sugar levels and keep them in the target range, among other things. To effectively manage your blood sugar level, you should balance what you drink and eat.

What you eat, how much you eat, and your timing is crucial in managing your blood sugar levels. The answer to all this is what I will share with you here.

22.   Macronutrients

When talking about healthy living, we can't proceed without mentioning macronutrients. So what are they?

Macronutrients are also called macros. They are nutrients our body needs in large quantities to function properly. The nutrients provide your body with energy measured in kcals or calories. There are three types of macronutrients:

Carbohydrates

Carbohydrates supply energy to the body. They are broken down into glucose and monosaccharides. Carbohydrates are not equal; they are either simple or complex.

Simple carbohydrates: These comprise small molecules that are digested easily and are responsible for a rapid increase in glucose levels.

Complex carbohydrates: Unlike the simple ones, larger molecules are broken down into smaller molecules. They take time to digest and are slow in increasing blood sugar.

The rapid consumption of carbohydrates will increase plasma glucose levels, which is measured by a glycemic index. Eating carbohydrates with a high glycemic index can easily increase your blood sugar glucose. On the other hand, eating foods with a low glycemic load will slowly increase your plasma glucose level.

Protein

Protein supplies the body with amino acids; the functions of the brain, blood, nervous system, hair, and skin are all made up of amino acids. It's also in charge of carrying oxygen and other vital nutrients all over the body. When carbohydrates and glucose are not available, the body will reverse-process protein to have energy.

Your body can make 11 amino acids on its own and get the other nine that it can't make through diet.

There are two types of protein, animal-based, and plant-based. Examples of plant-based proteins are seeds, nuts, and grains. The most common sources of protein can be sourced from meat, seafood products, eggs, and dairy.

According to the USDA, the daily requirements of protein sources should be anywhere from 10% to 30% of your daily calories.

Fats

Generally, people see fat as bad and try to avoid it in their diet. However, dietary fat is important in your journey of maintaining your sugar level low. Good fats protect your organs, allow proper cell function, and are also important for insulin. In terms of caloric deprivation or starving, fat can be a source of energy.

While good fats are crucial for a healthy diet, bad fats can gradually contribute to obesity. To maintain a healthy weight, fats should be consumed in moderation. Let's quickly take a look at the different types of fats.

Saturated fats: Saturated fats come from dairy sources and meat. When at room temperature, they are solid and can be shelf-stable for a while.

Unsaturated fats: These are good fats that are either monounsaturated or polyunsaturated. They come from meat and some plant sources and are very beneficial. They are liquid under normal room temperature and remain so even after refrigeration. They have a shorter shelf life than saturated fats.

Trans Fats: These are polyunsaturated fats that change from liquid to solid form and are extremely unhealthy for you. They are used in processed food, fast food, cakes, cookies, and any other food that contains hydrogenated fats.

23.   Other Essential Nutrients

Besides macros, which provide your body with nutrients, there are other essential nutrients you need to consider. These nutrients are also essential and need to be included in your diet.

Vitamin D

Vitamin D is a little deliberated fat-soluble hormone that provides many benefits. It helps in maintaining joints, bones, teeth and boosts the immune system. Examples of foods you can get the vitamin from include nuts, eggs, seeds, butter, and oily fish.

Additionally, by exposing yourself to the sun for 30 minutes daily, you encourage your vitamin D production and reduce your risk for diabetes.

Magnesium

This is a must-have nutrient in your diet. Research has suggested that people with Type 2 diabetes are more likely to have a deficiency in magnesium. Intracellular magnesium is responsible for vascular tone, regulating insulin's actions, and insulin-mediated glucose uptake. So, being deficient in magnesium isn't good, as it can worsen insulin resistance. Correcting a deficiency in magnesium will greatly help you manage your condition better.

Sodium

The function of sodium in the body is to transmit nerve pulses and control the electric charge both inside and outside your cells. When we eat mostly processed foods, we are most likely to consume more sodium than we want. Even though a high sodium intake is bad, a low intake can affect insulin resistance and cause cardiovascular disease.

The American Dietary Guidelines suggested that a daily intake of 2,300 milligrams shouldn't be exceeded. If you can, limit it to 1,500 milligrams; the lesser, the better.

24.   Recommended Nutrients for Diabetics

Nutrition is a crucial aspect that needs to be deliberated when treating diabetes. What goes into your system is part of what determines your blood sugar level. To maintain a proper blood sugar level, you need to pay attention to what you eat. Therefore, I will be sharing with you the recommended nutrients for diabetes. These are healthy foods you should stock your kitchen with.

Vegetables

- Carrots
- Broccoli
- Tomatoes
- Green peas
- Green pepper

Fruits

- Berries (strawberries, blueberries, blackberries)

- Oranges

- Citrus

- Apples

- Grapes

Grains (whole grains)

- Oats

- Quinoa

- Barley

- Cornmeal

- Brown rice

Dairy: low-fat

- Yogurt

- Milk

- Cheese

- Almond milk, soy milk

Protein

- Turkey or chicken without skin

- Lean meat

- Eggs

- Fish

- Nuts

- Split peas

- Chickpeas

- Dried beans

- Meat substitutes (tofu)

The foods you can eat are not limited to my suggestions above. There are other healthy foods you can eat. Instead of stick margarine, shortening, and lard, make use of oils when cooking. Also, make sure you include foods with heart-healthy fats in your diet. Some of these include avocado, olive oil, canola, nuts and seeds, tuna, salmon, and mackerel.

Each nutrient has its specific roles in the body. Since you are managing a health condition, you need to balance them to avoid loading yourself up with excess carbs. A diabetic diet will help you figure out how to balance nutrients and make healthy choices.

25.   Watch What You Eat

Watching what you eat is one of the things to do when controlling your blood sugar. The starches and sugars in your food significantly impact your body; this makes it very important to know what you are eating. To support this, there are some steps to take, and I have highlighted them below.

26.   Learn Portion Control

Portion control entails choosing a healthy size of certain foods. To effectively control your blood sugar, you need to be in control of the food you eat. Portion control can help you lose weight, digest food easily, stay energized, and reduce the intake of problematic foods. According to the (ADA) American Diabetes Association, your plate should have a lesser portion of starch and lean meats and a bigger portion of non-starchy vegetables.

27.   Limit Some Foods and Drinks

Below are some foods and drinks you should limit to support your healthy eating journey.

- Foods high in sodium
- Sweets (ice cream, baked goods, and candy)
- Fried foods high in trans-fat and saturated fat
- Beverages with added sugar (soda, energy drinks, and juice)

I would advise you to drink water instead of drinking sweetened beverages. Also, consider using a sugar substitute for your food. Examples of healthy sugar substitutes include tagatose, stevia, neotame, and acesulfame potassium. Avoid aspartame and sucralose, which are not healthy.

If you can avoid drinking alcohol, please do. However, if you must drink, it should be in moderate quantities. Men shouldn't drink more than two drinks, and women shouldn't go beyond one drink. Alcohol can make your blood sugar level low or too high; it's best to be avoided. Also, avoid carb-rich drinks, like wine and beer.

CHAPTER 7. BREAKFAST RECIPES

1. Coconut Pancake

Preparation time: 5 minutes

Cooking time: 15 minutes

Servings: 4

Ingredients:

- 1 cup coconut flour
- 2 tbsp. arrowroot powder
- 1 tsp. baking powder
- 1 cup coconut milk
- 3 tbsp. coconut oil

Directions:

1. In a medium container, mix the dry ingredients all together.
2. Add the coconut milk and a couple of tbsp. of copra oil, then mix properly.
3. In a skillet, melt 1 tsp. of copra oil.
4. Pour a ladle of the batter into the skillet, then swirl the pan to spread the batter evenly into a smooth pancake.
5. Cook it for like 3 minutes on medium heat until it becomes firm.
6. Turn the pancake to the other side, then cook it for an additional 2 minutes until it turns golden brown.
7. Cook the remaining pancakes in the same process.
8. Serve.

Nutrition:

- Calories: 377
- Carbohydrates: 60.7 g
- Protein: 6.4 g
- Fat: 14.9 g

2. Quinoa Porridge

Preparation time: 5 minutes

Cooking time: 25 minutes

Servings: 2

Ingredients:

- 2 cups coconut milk
- 1 cup rinsed quinoa
- 1/8 tsp. ground cinnamon
- 1 cup fresh blueberries

Directions:

1. In a saucepan, boil the coconut milk over high heat.
2. Add the quinoa to the milk, then allow the mixture to boil.

3. You then let it simmer for a quarter-hour on medium heat until the milk is reduced.

4. Add the cinnamon, then mix it properly in the saucepan.

5. Cover the saucepan and cook for at least 8 minutes until the milk is absorbed.

6. Add in the blueberries, then cook for 30 more seconds.

7. Serve.

Nutrition:

- Calories: 271
- Carbohydrates: 54 g
- Protein: 6.5 g
- Fat: 3.7 g

3. Amaranth Porridge

Preparation time: 5 minutes

Cooking time: 30 minutes

Servings: 2.

Ingredients:

- 2 cups coconut milk
- 2 cups alkaline water
- 1 cup amaranth
- 2 tbsp. coconut oil
- 1 tbsp. ground cinnamon

Directions:

1. In a saucepan, mix the milk with water, then boil the mixture.

2. You stir in the amaranth, then reduce the heat to medium.

3. Cook on medium heat, then simmer for at least half-hour as you stir it occasionally.

4. Close up the heat.

5. Add in cinnamon and copra oil, then stir.

6. Serve.

Nutrition:

- Calories: 434
- Carbohydrates: 27 g
- Protein: 6.7 g
- Fat: 35 g

4. Overnight Oatmeal with Berries and Nuts

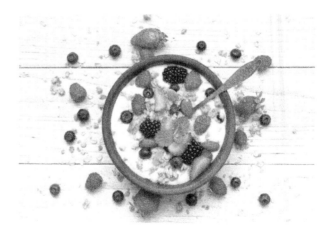

Preparation time: 5 minutes

Cooking time: 0 minute

Servings: 1

Ingredients:

- 1/2 medium-size ripe banana
- 1/8 tsp. kosher salt
- 2/3 cup unsweetened almond milk
- 1/4 cup frozen-thawed mixed berries
- 1 tbsp. chopped walnuts
- 1/4 cup plain 2% reduced-fat Greek yogurt
- 1/2 cup old-fashioned rolled oats
- 1 tsp. chia seeds

Directions:

1. In a small bowl, place the banana, and use a fork to mash it thoroughly.
2. Add yogurt and mix to combine.
3. Add chia seeds, oats, salt, and almond milk.
4. Mix well and cover.
5. Refrigerate over the night or at least 6 hours.
6. Top with mixed berries and walnuts.
7. Serve and enjoy.

Nutrition:

- Calories: 359
- Protein: 14 g
- Fat: 13 g
- Saturated fat: 2 g
- Sugar: 14 g
- Fiber: 10 g
- Sodium: 397 mg
- Calcium: 26% DV
- Potassium: 16% DV

5. Mushroom Breakfast Burrito

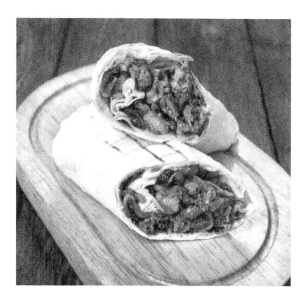

Preparation time: 10 minutes

Cooking time: 20 minutes

Servings: 1

Ingredients:

- 1/2 tbsp. neutral oil canola, vegetable, grape-seed
- 1/8 white onion diced
- 1/2 garlic clove minced
- 1/2 cups Cremini mushrooms chopped
- Cooking spray
- 1 large whole wheat tortillas
- 2/3 cup + 2 tbsp. goat cheese
- 1 cups loosely packed spinach chopped
- 2/3 tsp. salt
- 2 large eggs

- 3/4 tbsp. milk
- Salt and pepper to taste

Directions:

1. Add oil to the pan in a large skillet over medium-high heat.
2. Add the garlic, onion and cook until translucent, for about 2 to 3 minutes. Add the mushrooms, then cook for 3 minutes until they are golden brown.
3. Flip the mushrooms to allow the other side to cook.
4. In the pan, place spinach and cook for about 3 to 4 minutes until it's wilted. Season with salt and stir all the veggies together. Remove from the heat, then set it aside.
5. Whisk together milk and eggs in a large bowl. Season with pepper and salt to taste.
6. Over medium heat, heat another large skillet, spray the skillet using cooking spray. Add egg mixture, then cook until the eggs have set, frequently stirring, for about 4 to 5 minutes. Remove from heat.
7. In the microwave, heat the tortillas for 10 seconds.
8. On a piece of aluminum foil, lay out the tortillas and spread half tbsp. of goat cheese on it.
9. Distribute the roasted vegetables and scrambled eggs evenly.
10. Roll up in the foil and place it in a freezer bag. Then freeze.
11. Unwrap the burritos from the foil when ready to eat from the freezer. Serve and enjoy.

Nutrition:

- Calories: 385
- Protein: 20 g
- Fat: 22 g
- Saturated fat: 6 g
- Sugar: 4 g
- Fiber: 4 g
- Sodium: 640 mg
- Calcium: 21% DV
- Potassium: 487 mg

6. No-Bake Blueberry Oats Bites

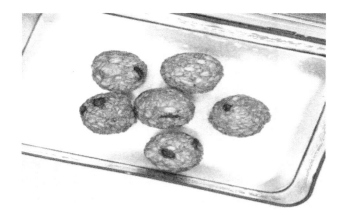

Preparation time: 10 minutes

Cooking time: 0 minutes

Servings: 1

Ingredients:

- 1 cup old-fashioned rolled
- 2/3 cup packed Medjool dates, pitted and chopped (about 7–8 large ones)
- 1 tsp. vanilla extract
- A pinch of salt
- 1–3 tbsp. water, as needed
- 1/2 cup dried blueberries
- 1 tsp. fresh lemon juice

Directions:

1. In your food processor, add all the ingredients together.
2. Wait and scrape down the sides as needed. Do this until it's well-combined.
3. Add more water if you want to get the mixture to come together.
4. Roll mixture into golf ball-sized cookie balls.
5. Serve immediately or cover and refrigerate.
6. Enjoy!

Nutrition:

- Calories: 101
- Protein: 0 g
- Fat: 0 g
- Saturated fat: 0 g
- Sugar: 13 g
- Fiber: 1 g
- Sodium: 14 mg
- Calcium: 0% DV
- Potassium: 0% DV

7. Avocado and Egg on Whole Wheat Toast

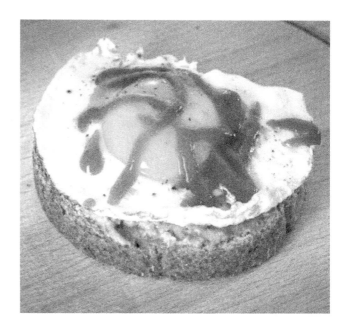

Preparation time: 5 minutes

Cooking time: 0 minutes

Servings: 1

Ingredients:

- 1/4 avocado
- 1 slice whole-wheat bread, toasted
- 1 large egg, fried
- 1/4 tsp. ground pepper
- 1/8 tsp. garlic powder

Directions:

1. Combine pepper, avocado, and garlic powder in a small bowl.
2. Gently mash together.

3. Top the toast with the avocado mixture and fried egg.
4. Serve and enjoy.

Nutrition:

- Calories: 270.9
- Protein: 11.5 g
- Fat: 17.7 g
- Saturated fat: 3.5 g
- Sugar: 2 g
- Fiber: 5.4 g
- Sodium: 216.2 mg
- Calcium: 69.4 mg
- Potassium: 406.5 mg

8. A Cup of Cottage Cheese with Peach Slices

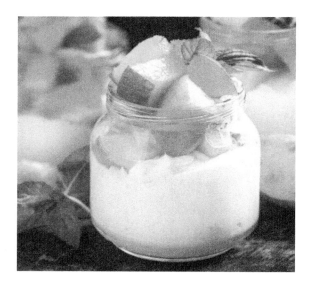

Preparation time: 3 minutes

Cooking time: 0 minutes

Servings: 1

Ingredients:

- 1 cup cottage cheese, low-fat
- 1 medium raw peaches

Directions:

1. Cut the peach in half.
2. Remove pit.
3. Cut peach into bite-size pieces.
4. Mix with cottage cheese.
5. Serve yourself and enjoy it.

Nutrition:

- Calories: 221
- Protein: 29g
- Fat: 1.5 g
- Saturated fat: 1.5 g
- Sugar: 18.7 g
- Fiber: 2.3 g
- Sodium: 917.6 mg
- Calcium: 146.8 mg
- Potassium: 479.4 mg

9. Peanut Butter Sandwich with Strawberry Jam

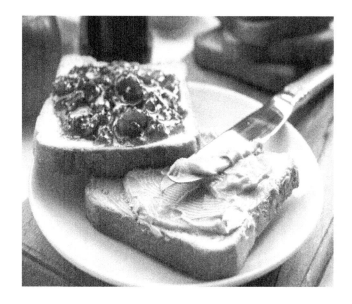

Preparation time: 5 minutes

Cooking time: 0 minutes

Servings: 1

Ingredients:

- 1 tbsp. strawberry jam
- 1 tbsp. peanut butter
- 1 slice whole-grain sandwich bread (toasted)

Directions:

1. Spread peanut butter on the sandwich first using a knife before you add the jam.
2. Add the jam.
3. Serve and enjoy.

Nutrition:

- Calories: 193
- Protein: 7g
- Fat: 83 g
- Saturated fat: 2 g
- Sugar: 8 g
- Fiber: 2 g
- Sodium: 205.88 mg
- Calcium: 45.77 mg
- Potassium: 178.63 mg

10. Chicken Nacho Casserole

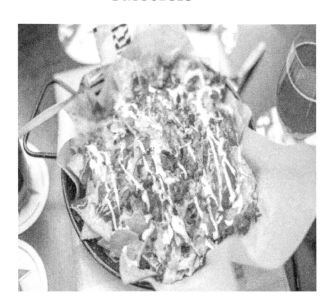

Preparation time: 5 minutes

Cooking time: 25 minutes

Servings: 1

Ingredients:

- 1 non-stick cooking spray
- 2 tsp. chili powder
- 1/2 tsp. cumin
- 1/2 tsp. garlic powder
- 2/3 cup cheddar cheese (reduced-fat, shredded)
- 1/8 tsp. black pepper
- 1 lb. chicken breasts (boneless, skinless, cut into small pieces)
- 1 can fire-roasted tomatoes (15 oz., diced)
- 1 cup black beans (no salt added, drained and rinsed)
- 1 1/2 oz. baked tortilla chips (crushed, (or about 24)

Directions:

1. Preheat the oven to 375°F.
2. Use cooking spray to spray a 2 1/2 qt. baking dish.
3. Season the chicken with black pepper.
4. Use cooking spray to spray a large sauté pan and heat over medium-high.
5. Add the chicken. Then cook for about 8 minutes.
6. Add the black beans, diced tomatoes, chili powder, garlic powder, and cumin to the pan.
7. Reduce the heat to low. Then simmer for about 5 minutes.
8. Pour the chicken mixture into the baking dish.
9. Sprinkle cheese on top. Then top with the crushed tortilla chips.

10. Bake until the cheese is melted for about 12 minutes.

Nutrition:

- Calories: 210
- Protein: 23 g
- Fat: 6 g
- Saturated fat: 2.5 g
- Sugar: 3 g
- Fiber: 3 g
- Sodium: 360 mg
- Calcium: 0 mg
- Potassium: 460 mg

11. Stir-Fried Vegetable and Egg Omelet

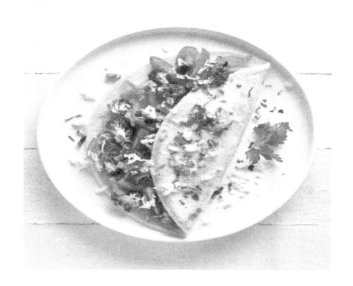

Preparation time: 5 minutes

Cooking time: 25 minutes

Servings: 1

Ingredients:

- 1/2 cup no-salt-added diced tomatoes with garlic, basil, and oregano, well-drained
- 1/2 cup cucumber, chopped and seeded
- 1/2 cup f chopped yellow summer squash
- 1/2 ripe avocado, pitted, peeled, and chopped
- 1/4 tsp. ground black pepper
- 1 Non-stick cooking spray
- 1/4 cup shredded reduced-fat Monterey Jack cheese with jalapeño Chile peppers
- 2 eggs
- 1 cup refrigerated or frozen egg product, thawed
- 2 tbsp. water
- 1 tsp. dried basil, crushed
- 1/4 tsp. salt

Directions:

1. Stir together cucumber, tomatoes, squash, and avocado in a medium bowl. Set it aside. Whisk together eggs, water, egg product, salt, basil, and pepper in a medium bowl.
2. For the Omelet, use cooking spray to coat an 8-inch non-stick skillet generously. Heat skillet over medium heat, and add 1/3 cup of the egg mixture into the hot skillet.
3. Use a spatula to start stirring the eggs gently but continuously until the mixture resembles cooked egg pieces surrounded by liquid egg. Stop stirring and cook until the egg is set but shiny for about 30 to 60 seconds.
4. Spoon a half cup of the filling over one side of the Omelet, and carefully fold Omelet over the filling. Carefully remove Omelet from the skillet and repeat to make as much Omelet as you can eat.
5. Use paper towels to wipe the skillet clean, then spray with cooking spray between omelets.
6. Sprinkle 1 tbsp. cheese over each Omelet.
7. Serve yourself and enjoy it.

Nutrition:

- Calories: 128.2
- Protein: 12.3 g
- Fat: 6.1 g
- Saturated fat: 1.9 g
- Sugar: 4.1 g
- Fiber: 3.5 g
- Sodium: 357.5 mg
- Calcium: 120 mg
- Potassium: 341.1 mg

12. Banana and Berry Smoothie

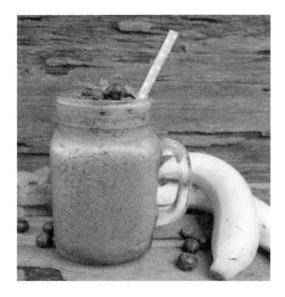

Preparation time: 5 minutes

Cooking time: 0 minutes

Servings: 1

Ingredients:

- 1/2 cup frozen blueberries
- 1 tsp. honey
- 1/8 tsp. vanilla extract
- 1/3 cup rolled oats
- 1 tbsp. chia seeds
- 1/2 banana
- 1/3 cup plain Greek yogurt
- 1/3 cup milk
- 1/4 cup chopped walnuts, divided

Directions:

1. Place the banana, blueberries, milk, yogurt, honey, 3 tbsp. walnuts, and vanilla in a blender.
2. Blend until smooth.
3. In a bowl, pour the blueberry-walnut mixture.
4. Stir in the chia seeds and oats.
5. Pour the mixture in a small serving container or in a jar.
6. Top with the rest of the walnuts.
7. Cover and refrigerate over the night, for about 4 hours.
8. Serve cold straight from the refrigerator.
9. Enjoy.

Nutrition:

- Calories: 514
- Protein: 20 g
- Fat: 24 g
- Saturated fat: 15 g
- Sugar: 0 g
- Fiber: 12 g
- Sodium: 69 mg
- Cholesterol: 10 mg

13. Make-Ahead Breakfast Quiche

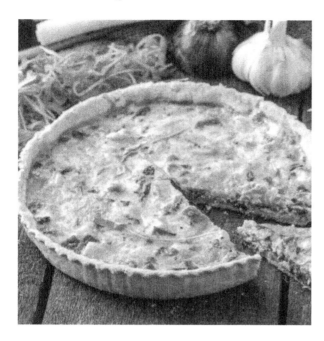

Preparation time: 15 minutes

Cooking time: 30 minutes

Servings: 1

Ingredients:

- 1 (9 inches) frozen whole-wheat pie-crust shell
- 1 (8 oz.) package of microwavable fresh broccoli florets
- 3 oz. sharp Cheddar cheese, shredded (about 3/4 cup)
- 3/4 tsp. kosher salt
- 1/4 tsp. black pepper
- 1 1/2 tsp. olive oil
- 1 cup chopped sweet onion (from 1 large onion)
- 4 large eggs
- 1/2 cup evaporated milk

Directions:

1. Preheat oven to 400°F.
2. Let the pie-crust thaw for about 10 minutes at room temperature.
3. Place in the preheated oven, and bake for about 10 to 15 minutes, until lightly browned.
4. Let it cool for about 10 minutes.
5. Reduce oven temperature to 375°F.
6. Cook broccoli according to package instruction, for about 3 minutes, until tender-crisp. Chop larger pieces coarsely.
7. In a large skillet, heat oil over medium-high and add onion. Cook for 10 minutes, until lightly golden.
8. Whisk together evaporated milk and eggs in a medium bowl.
9. Stir in cheese, broccoli, onion, black pepper, and salt.
10. Pour mixture into prepared pie crust.
11. Bake until just set and edges are golden brown at 375°F.
12. Serve and enjoy.

Nutrition:

- Calories: 231
- Protein: 10 g

- Fat: 16 g
- Saturated fat: 8 g
- Sugar: 3 g
- Fiber: 3 g
- Sodium: 404 mg
- Calcium: 150 mg
- Potassium: 204 mg

14. Cheesy Ham and Hash Casserole

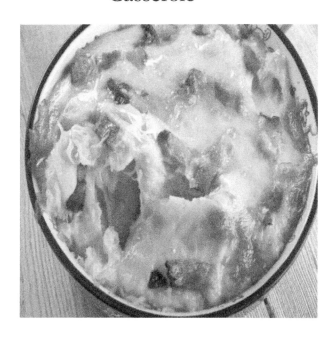

Preparation time: 15 minutes

Cooking time: 1 hour

Servings: 1

Ingredients:

- 1/8 (10.75 oz.) can have condensed cream of potato soup
- 1/8 (16 oz.) container of sour cream
- 2 tbsp. + 3/4 tsp. shredded sharp Cheddar cheese
- 1/8 (32 oz.) package of frozen Hash Brown potatoes
- 1/2 oz. cooked, diced ham
- 1 tbsp. + 1 3/4 tsp. grated Parmesan cheese

Directions:

1. Preheat oven to 375°F.
2. Grease a 9x13-inch baking dish lightly.
3. Mix hash browns, the cream of potato soup, ham, Cheddar cheese, and sour cream together in a large bowl.
4. Spread evenly into the prepared dish.
5. Sprinkle with Parmesan cheese.
6. Bake for about an hour in the preheated oven, or until lightly brown and bubbly.
7. Serve immediately.
8. Enjoy.

Nutrition:

- Calories: 414.6
- Protein: 14.4 g
- Fat: 27.2 g
- Saturated fat: 14.7 g
- Sugar: 0.7 g
- Fiber: 2.4 g
- Sodium: 760.6 mg
- Calcium: 304.1 mg
- Potassium: 437.8 mg

15. Egg and Bacon Tacos

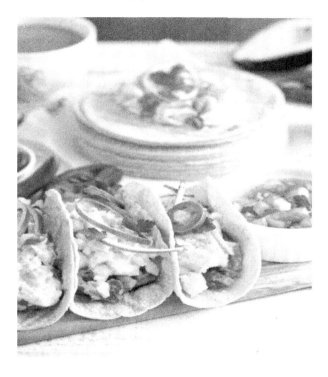

Preparation time: 5 minutes

Cooking time: 3 minutes

Servings: 1

Ingredients:

- 1 egg
- 1/8 tsp. salt
- 1/8 tsp. ground black pepper
- 1 flour tortillas
- 2 tsp. crumbled cooked bacon
- 1 tsp. butter
- 1/2 slice of American cheese, diced
- 2 tbsp. + 2 tsp. salsa (optional)

Directions:

1. In a bowl, whisk eggs together and stir in bacon.
2. In a skillet over medium heat, melt butter and add the egg mixture.
3. Cook and stir for about 2 to 3 minutes, until eggs are completely set.
4. Stir in American cheese, pepper, and salt.
5. Wrap tortillas in damp paper towels; microwave for about a minute, until warmed through.
6. Spoon 1/8 cup egg mixture into the center of the tortilla.
7. Fold sides to cover.
8. Serve with salsa.
9. Enjoy.

Nutrition:

- Calories: 435.7
- Protein: 18.9 g
- Fat: 22 g
- Saturated fat: 9.2 g
- Sugar: 3.2 g
- Fiber: 2.9 g
- Sodium: 1295.4 mg
- Calcium: 211.7 mg
- Potassium: 375.4 mg

16. Breakfast Crepes

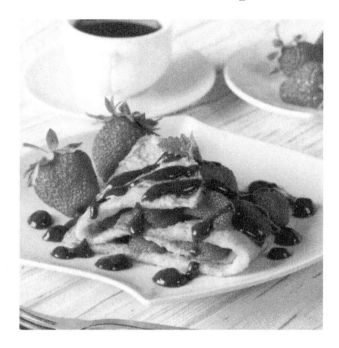

Preparation time: 10 minutes

Cooking time: 20 minutes

Servings: 1

Ingredients:

- 1/4 cup all-purpose flour
- 2 tbsp. milk
- 2 tbsp. water
- 1/8 tsp. salt
- 1/2 eggs
- 1 1/2 tsp. butter, melted

Directions:

1. Whisk together the eggs and flour in a large mixing bowl.

2. Gradually add in the water and milk, stirring to combine.

3. Add the butter and salt; beat until smooth.

4. Bring a lightly oiled frying pan over medium-high heat.

5. Pour or scoop the batter onto the griddle, using approx. 1/4 cup of each of the crepe.

6. Tilt the pan with a circular motion so the batter will coat the surface evenly.

7. Cook the crepe until the bottom is brown lightly for about 2 minutes.

8. Loosen with a spatula.

9. Turn and cook the other side.

10. Serve hot and enjoy.

Nutrition:

- Calories: 215.7
- Protein: 7.4 g
- Fat: 9.2 g
- Saturated fat: 4.9 g
- Sugar: 1.7 g
- Fiber: 0.8 g
- Sodium: 235.5 mg
- Calcium: 56.3 mg
- Potassium: 114.7 mg

17. No-Bake Nut Butter Protein Bites

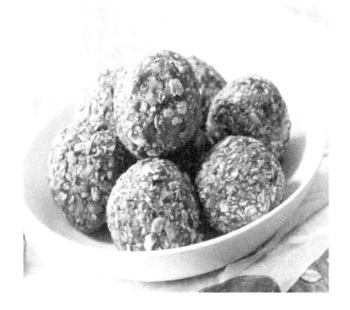

Preparation time: 10 minutes

Cooking time: 20 minutes

Servings: 1

Ingredients:

- 1 cup old-fashioned oats
- 1/8 tsp. sea salt
- 1/2 cup creamy peanut butter
- 1/4 cup honey
- 1/4 cup ground flax seed
- 1 tsp. vanilla extract
- 1/4 tsp. ground cinnamon
- 1 tbsp. chia seeds
- 1/4 cup semi-sweet chocolate chips

Directions:

1. In a large mixing bowl, add all ingredients together, and combine.
2. Cover using plastic wrap or a lid.
3. Place the mixture inside the refrigerator for about 30 minutes (this will help in making them easier to roll)
4. Roll into your desired amount of bites using 2 tbsp. the scooper.
5. Store in the refrigerator in an airtight container for up to 7 days. You can freeze for up to 3 months as well.
6. Serve and enjoy.

Nutrition:

- Calories: 155
- Protein: 4 g
- Fat: 9 g
- Saturated fat: 2 g
- Sugar: 8 g
- Fiber: 2 g
- Sodium: 75 mg
- Calcium: 25 mg
- Potassium: 150 mg

18. Chicken on Whole Wheat Toast with Olive Oil

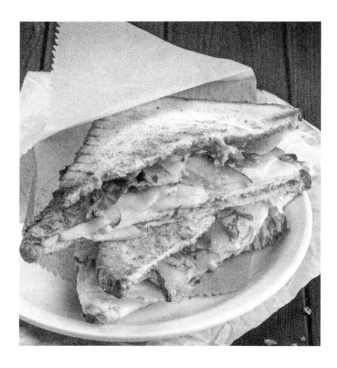

Preparation time: 5 minutes

Cooking time: 5 minutes

Servings: 1

Ingredients:

- 1 tbsp. light mayonnaise
- 1 slice (about 1 oz.) of crusty whole-wheat bread
- 1/4 cup fresh tarragon
- 1 piece of reduced-fat Swiss cheese
- 4 oz. cooked chicken breast
- 1/8 tsp. salt
- 1/8 tsp. black pepper
- 1/2 olive oil spray

Directions:

1. Spread mayonnaise on the bread.
2. Top with the tarragon, chicken, and cheese.
3. Sprinkle with pepper and salt, then top with the rest of the slices of bread.
4. Coat a non-stick skillet with olive oil spray.
5. Heat over low heat.
6. Add the sandwich and press down using a lid or any other clean pan.
7. Cook for about 2 minutes, flip and press again. Cook for another 2 minutes.
8. Cut the sandwich in half.
9. Serve with salad and enjoy it.

Nutrition:

- Calories: 240
- Protein: 28 g
- Fat: 9 g
- Saturated fat: 3 g
- Sugar: 2 g
- Fiber: 2 g
- Sodium: 330 mg
- Potassium: 250 mg

19. Egg and Avocado Omelet

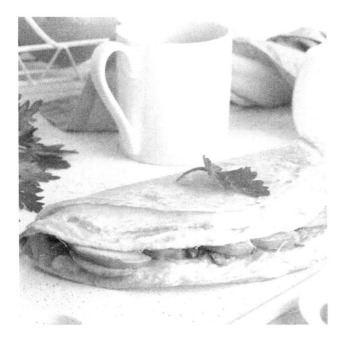

Preparation time: 15 minutes

Cooking time: 8 minutes

Servings: 1

Ingredients:

- 3 large eggs
- 1/4 cup chopped kalamata olives
- 1 tbsp. chopped fresh basil
- 3/4 cup feta cheese
- 1/2 avocado, diced
- 1/2 cup diced tomatoes

Directions:

1. In a small bowl, whisk eggs until smooth.
2. Preheat a non-stick skillet over medium heat.
3. Pour in eggs and scatter avocado, feta cheese, olives, tomatoes, and basil over 1 side.
4. Cook for about 5 minutes until the bottom is golden brown.
5. Fold over; cook for about 3 minutes, until the center is set.
6. Serve and enjoy.

Nutrition:

- Calories: 392
- Protein: 19.1 g
- Fat: 31.3 g
- Saturated fat: 12.3 g
- Sugar: 4.4 g
- Fiber: 4.1 g
- Sodium: 113.6 mg
- Calcium: 335.9 mg
- Potassium: 489.6 mg

20. Apple and Cinnamon Overnight Oats

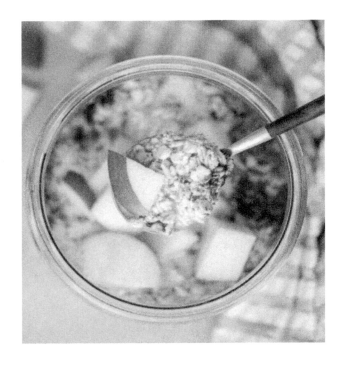

Preparation time: 10 minutes

Cooking time: 0 minutes

Servings: 1

Ingredients:

- 1/2 cup old-fashioned rolled oats
- 1/4 tsp. ground cinnamon
- A pinch of salt
- 1/2 cup diced apple
- 1/2 cup unsweetened almond milk
- 1/2 tbsp. chia seeds
- 1 tsp. maple syrup
- 2 tbsp. toasted pecans

Directions:

1. Combine almond milk, oats, chia seeds (if using), cinnamon, maple syrup, and salt in a pint-sized jar.
2. Stir together.
3. Cover and refrigerate over the night.
4. Before serving, top with pecans and apple, if you feel like.
5. Serve and enjoy.

Nutrition:

- Calories: 215
- Protein: 5.8 g
- Fat: 4.4 g
- Saturated fat: 0.5 g
- Sugar: 11.3 g
- Fiber: 6.3 g
- Sodium: 231.8 mg
- Calcium: 262 mg
- Potassium: 248.9 mg

21. Country-Style Pork Ribs

Preparation Time: 5 minutes

Cooking Time: 20−25 minutes

Servings: 4

Ingredients:

- 12 country-style pork ribs, trimmed excess fat
- 2 tbsp. cornstarch
- 2 tbsp. olive oil
- 1 tsp. dry mustard
- 1/2 tsp. thyme
- 1/2 tsp. garlic powder
- 1 tsp. dried marjoram
- Pinch salt
- Freshly ground black pepper, to taste

Directions:

1. Place the ribs on a clean work surface.
2. In a small bowl, combine the cornstarch, olive oil, mustard, thyme, garlic powder, marjoram, salt, and pepper, and rub into the ribs.
3. Place the ribs in the air fryer basket and roast at 400°F (204°C) for 10 minutes.
4. Carefully, turn the ribs using tongs and roast for 10 to 15 minutes or until the ribs are crisp and register an internal temperature of at least 150°F (66°C).

Nutrition:

- Calories: 579
- Fat: 44 g
- Protein: 40 g
- Carbs: 4 g
- Fiber: 0 g
- Sugar: 0 g
- Sodium: 155 mg

22. Lemon and Honey Pork Tenderloi

Preparation Time: 5 minutes

Cooking Time: 10 minutes

Servings: 4

Ingredients:

- 1 (1 pound/454 g) pork tenderloin, cut into ½-inch slices
- 1 tbsp. olive oil
- 1 tbsp. freshly squeezed lemon juice
- 1 tbsp. honey
- 1/2 tsp. grated lemon zest
- 1/2 tsp. dried marjoram
- Pinch salt
- Freshly ground black pepper to taste

Directions:

1. Put the pork tenderloin slices in a medium bowl.
2. In a small bowl, combine the olive oil, lemon juice, honey, lemon zest, marjoram, salt, and pepper. Mix.
3. Pour this marinade over the tenderloin slices and massage gently with your hands to work it into the pork.

4. Place the pork in the air fryer basket and roast at 400°F (204°C) for 10 minutes or until the pork registers at least 145°F (63°C) using a meat thermometer.

Nutrition:

- Calories: 208
- Fat: 8 g
- Protein: 30 g
- Carbs: 5 g
- Fiber: 0 g
- Sugar: 4 g
- Sodium: 104 mg

23. Dijon Pork Tenderloin

Preparation Time: 10 minutes

Cooking Time: 12−14 minutes

Servings: 4

Ingredients:

- 1 lb. (454 g) pork tenderloin, cut into 1-inch slices
- Pinch salt
- Freshly ground black pepper to taste
- 2 tbsp. Dijon mustard
- 1 garlic clove, minced
- 1/2 tsp. dried basil
- 1 cup soft bread crumbs
- 2 tbsp. olive oil

Directions:

1. Slightly pound the pork slices until they are about ¾ inch thick. Sprinkle with salt and pepper on both sides.
2. Coat the pork with the Dijon mustard and sprinkle with garlic and basil.
3. On a plate, combine the bread crumbs and olive oil and mix well. Coat the pork slices with the bread crumb mixture, patting, so the crumbs adhere.
4. Place the pork in the air fryer basket, leaving a little space between each piece. Air fry at 390°F (199°C) for 12 to 14 minutes or until the pork reaches at least 145°F (63°C) on a meat thermometer, and the coating is crisp and brown. Serve immediately.

Nutrition:

- Calories: 336
- Fat: 13 g
- Protein: 34 g
- Carbs: 20 g
- Fiber: 2 g
- Sugar: 2 g
- Sodium: 390 mg

24. Pork Satay

Preparation Time: 15 minutes

Cooking Time: 9−14 minutes

Servings: 4

Ingredients:

- 1 (1 lb. / 454 g) pork tenderloin, cut into 1½-inch cubes
- 1/4 cup minced onion
- 2 garlic cloves, minced
- 1 jalapeño pepper, minced
- 2 tbsp. freshly squeezed lime juice
- 2 tbsp. coconut milk
- 2 tbsp. unsalted peanut butter
- 2 tsp. curry powder

Directions:

1. In a medium bowl, mix the pork, onion, garlic, jalapeño, lime juice, coconut milk, peanut butter, and curry powder until well combined. Let stand for 10 minutes at room temperature.
2. With a slotted spoon, remove the pork from the marinade. Reserve the marinade.
3. Thread the pork onto about 8 bamboo or metal skewers. Air fry at 380ºF (193ºC) for 9 to 14 minutes, brushing once with the reserved marinade until the pork reaches at least 145ºF (63ºC) on a meat thermometer. Discard any remaining marinade. Serve immediately.

Nutrition:

- Calories: 195
- Fat: 7 g
- Protein: 25 g
- Carbs: 7 g
- Fiber: 1 g
- Sugar: 3 g
- Sodium: 65 mg

25.   Pork Burgers with Red Cabbage Slaw

Preparation Time: 20 minutes

Cooking Time: 7−9 minutes

Servings: 4

Ingredients:

- 1/2 cup Greek yogurt
- 2 tbsp. low-sodium mustard, divided
- 1 tbsp. freshly squeezed lemon juice
- 1/4 cup sliced red cabbage
- 1/4 cup grated carrots
- 1 pound (454 g) lean ground pork
- 1/2 tsp. paprika
- 1 cup mixed baby lettuce greens
- 2 small tomatoes, sliced
- 8 small low-sodium whole-wheat sandwich buns, cut in half

Directions:

1. In a small bowl, combine the yogurt, 1 tablespoon mustard, lemon juice, cabbage, and carrots; mix and refrigerate.

2. In a medium bowl, combine the pork, the remaining 1 tablespoon mustard, and paprika. Form into 8 small patties.

3. Put the patties into the air fryer basket. Air fry at 400°F (204°C) for 7 to 9 minutes, or until the patties register 165°F (74°C) as tested with a meat thermometer.

4. Assemble the burgers by placing some of the lettuce greens on a bun bottom. Top with a tomato slice, the patties, and the cabbage mixture. Add the bun top and serve immediately.

Nutrition:

- Calories: 473
- Fat: 15 g
- Protein: 35 g
- Carbs: 51 g
- Fiber: 8 g
- Sugar: 8 g
- Sodium: 138 mg

26. Breaded Pork Chops

Preparation Time: 10 minutes

Cooking Time: 12 minutes

Servings: 4

Ingredients:

- 1 cup Whole-wheat breadcrumbs
- Salt ¼ tsp.
- 2–4 pcs. pork chops (center cut and boneless)
- 1/2 tsp. chili powder
- 1 tbsp. parmesan cheese
- 1½ tsp. paprika
- 1 egg beaten
- 1/2 tsp. onion powder
- 1/2 tsp. grounded garlic
- Pepper to taste

Directions:

1. Let the air fryer preheat to 400°F
2. Rub kosher salt on each side of pork chops, let it rest
3. Add beaten egg in a big bowl
4. Add Parmesan cheese, breadcrumbs, garlic, pepper, paprika, chili powder, and onion powder in a bowl and mix well
5. Dip pork chop in egg, then in breadcrumb mixture
6. Put it in the air fryer and spray it with oil.
7. Let it cook for 12 minutes at 400°F. Flip it over halfway through. Cook for another 6 minutes.
8. Serve with a side of salad.

Nutrition:

- Calories: 425
- Fat: 20 g
- Fiber: 5 g
- Protein: 31 g
- Carbs: 19 g

27.   Pork Taquitos in Air Fryer

Preparation Time: 10 minutes

Cooking Time: 7-10 minutes

Servings: 2

Ingredients:

- 3 cups pork tenderloin, cooked and shredded
- Cooking spray
- 2 ½ shredded mozzarella, fat-free
- 10 small tortillas
- 1 lime juice

Directions:

1. Let the air fryer preheat to 380°F.
2. Add lime juice to pork and mix well.
3. With a damp towel over the tortilla, microwave for 10 seconds to soften.
4. Add pork filling and cheese on top in a tortilla, roll up the tortilla tightly.
5. Place tortillas on a greased foil pan
6. Spray oil over tortillas. Cook for 7 to 10 minutes or until tortillas are golden brown, flip halfway through.
7. Serve with fresh salad.

Nutrition:

- Calories: 253
- Fat: 18 g
- Carbs: 10 g
- Protein: 20 g

28.   Tasty Egg Rolls

Preparation Time: 10 minutes

Cooking Time: 20 minutes

Servings: 3

Ingredients:

- 1/2 bag coleslaw mix
- 1/2 onion
- 1/2 tsp. salt
- 1/2 cup mushrooms
- Lean ground pork: 2 cups
- 1 stalk celery
- 12 Wrappers (egg roll)

Directions:

1. Put a skillet over medium flame, add onion and lean ground pork and cook for 5 to 7 minutes.
2. Add coleslaw mixture, salt, mushrooms, and celery to skillet and cook for almost 5 minutes.
3. Lay egg roll wrapper flat and add filling (1/3 cup), roll it up, seal with water.
4. Spray with oil the rolls.
5. Put in the air fryer for 6 to 8 minutes at 400°F, flipping once halfway through.
6. Serve hot.

Nutrition:

- Calories: 245
- Fat: 10 g
- Carbs: 9 g
- Protein: 11 g

29.   Pork Dumplings

Preparation Time: 30 minutes

Cooking Time: 20 minutes

Servings: 4

Ingredients:

- 18 dumpling wrappers
- 1 tsp. olive oil
- 4 cups bok choy (chopped)
- 2 tbsp. rice vinegar
- 1 tbsp. diced ginger
- 1/4 tsp. crushed red pepper
- 1 tbsp. diced garlic
- 1/2 cup lean ground pork
- Cooking spray
- 2 tsp. lite soy sauce
- 1/2 tsp. honey
- 1 tsp. Toasted sesame oil
- 1/8 cup finely chopped scallions

Directions:

1. Preheat the air fryer oven to 400°F (205°C).

2. Add bok choy, cook for 6 minutes, and add garlic, ginger, and cook for 1 minute. Move this mixture on a paper towel, and pat dry the excess oil

3. In a bowl, add bok choy mixture, crushed red pepper, and lean ground pork and mix well.

4. Lay a dumpling wrapper on a plate and add 1 tablespoon of filling in the wrapper's middle. With water, seal the edges and crimp them.

5. Spray oil on the air fryer basket, add dumplings in it and cook at 375°F for 12 minutes or until browned.

6. In the meantime, to make the sauce, add sesame oil, rice vinegar, scallions, soy sauce, and honey in a bowl mix together.

7. Serve the dumplings with sauce.

Nutrition:

- Calories: 140
- Fat: 5 g
- Protein: 12 g
- Carbs: 9 g

30.   Pork Chop & Broccoli

Preparation Time: 20 minutes

Cooking Time: 10 minutes

Servings: 2

Ingredients:

- 2 cups broccoli florets

- 2 pcs. bone-in pork chop
- 1/2 tsp. paprika
- 2 tbsp. avocado oil
- 1/2 tsp. garlic powder
- 1/2 tsp. onion powder
- 2 cloves crushed garlic
- 1 tsp. salt divided
- Cooking spray

Directions:

1. Let the air fryer preheat to 350°F. Spray the basket with cooking oil
2. Add 1 tablespoon avocado oil, onion powder, ½ teaspoon of salt, garlic powder, and paprika in a bowl, mix well, rub this spice mix to the pork chop's sides
3. Add pork chops to air fryer basket and let it cook for 5 minutes
4. In the meantime, add 1 remaining teaspoon of avocado oil, garlic, the other ½ teaspoon of salt, and broccoli to a bowl and coat well
5. Flip the pork chop and add the broccoli. Let it cook for 5 more minutes.
6. Take out from the air fryer and serve.

Nutrition:

- Calories: 483
- Fat: 20 g
- Carbs: 12 g
- Protein: 23 g

31.Cheesy Pork Chops

Preparation Time: 5 minutes

Cooking Time: 4 minutes

Servings: 2

Ingredients:

- 4 lean pork chops
- 1/2 tsp. salt
- 1/2 tsp. garlic powder
- 4 tbsp. shredded cheese
- 2 chopped cilantro

Directions:

1. Let the air fryer preheat to 350°F.
2. With garlic, cilantro, and salt, rub the pork chops. Put in the air fryer. Let it cook for 4 minutes.
3. Flip them and cook for 2 more minutes.
4. Add cheese on top of them and cook for another 2 minutes or until the cheese is melted.
5. Serve with salad greens.

Nutrition:

- Calories: 467
- Protein: 61 g
- Fat: 22 g
- Saturated Fat: 8 g

32.   Pork Rind Nachos

Preparation Time: 5 minutes

Cooking Time: 5 minutes

Servings: 2

Ingredients:

- 2 tbsp. pork rinds
- 1/4 cup shredded cooked chicken
- 1/2 cup shredded Monterey jack cheese
- 1/4 cup sliced pickled jalapeños
- 1/4 cup guacamole
- 1/4 cup full-fat sour cream

Directions:

1. Put pork rinds in a 6-inches round baking pan. Fill with grilled chicken and Monterey cheese jack. Place the pan in the basket with the air fryer.
2. Set the temperature to 370°F and set the timer for 5 minutes or until the cheese has been melted.
3. Eat right away with jalapeños, guacamole, and sour cream.

Nutrition:

- Calories: 295
- Protein: 30.1 g
- Fiber: 1.2 g
- Carbs: 1.8 g
- Fat: 27.5 g
- Carbs: 3.0 g

CHAPTER 8. VEGETARIAN BREAKFAST RECIPES

31. Eggplant Surprise

Preparation Time: 10−20 minutes

Cooking Time: 7 minutes

Servings: 4

Ingredients:

- 1 eggplant, roughly chopped
- 3 zucchinis, roughly chopped
- 3 tbsp. extra-virgin olive oil
- 3 tomatoes, sliced
- 2 tbsp. lemon juice
- 1 tsp. thyme, dried
- 1 tsp. oregano, dried
- Salt and black pepper to taste

Directions:

1. Put eggplant pieces in your air fryer oven.
2. Add zucchinis and tomatoes.
3. In a bowl, mix lemon juice with salt, pepper, thyme, oregano, and oil and stir well.
4. Pour this over veggie, toss to coat, seal the air fryer oven lid and cook at high for 7 minutes.
5. Quickly release the pressure, open the lid; divide among plates and serve.

Nutrition:

- Calories: 160
- Fat: 7 g
- Protein: 1 g
- Sugar: 6 g
- Carbs: 19 g
- Fiber: 8 g
- Sodium: 20 mg

32. Carrots and Turnips

Preparation Time: 10−20 minutes

Cooking Time: 9 minutes

Servings: 4

Ingredients:

- 2 turnips, peeled and sliced
- 1 small onion; chopped.
- 1 tsp. lemon juice
- 1 tsp. cumin, ground.
- 3 carrots, sliced
- 1 tbsp. extra-virgin olive oil
- 1 cup water
- Salt and black pepper to the taste

Directions:

1. Set your air fryer oven on "Sauté" mode; add oil and heat it.
2. Add onion, stir, and saute for 2 minutes.

3. Add turnips, carrots, cumin, and lemon juice, stir and cook for 1 minute.

4. Add salt, pepper, and water, then stir well. Close the lid and cook at high for 6 minutes.

5. Quickly release the pressure, open the air fryer oven lid, and divide turnips and carrots among plates and serve.

Nutrition:

- Calories: 170
- Fat: 9 g
- Protein: 1 g
- Sugar: 5 g
- Carbs: 19 g
- Fiber: 7 g
- Sodium: 475 mg

33.   Instant Brussels Sprouts with Parmesan

Preparation Time: 10−20 minutes

Cooking Time: 3 minutes

Servings: 4

Ingredients:

- 1 lb. brussels sprouts, washed
- 1 cup water
- 3 tbsp. Parmesan, grated
- 1 lemon juice
- 2 tbsp. butter
- Salt and black pepper to taste

Directions:

1. Put sprouts in your air fryer oven, add salt, pepper, and water; and then stir well. Close the lid and cook at high for 3 minutes.

2. Quickly release the pressure, transfer sprouts to a bowl, discard water and clean your pot.

3. Set your pot on "Sauté" mode; add butter and melt it.

4. Add lemon juice and stir well.

5. Add sprouts, stir and transfer to plates.

6. Add more salt, pepper if needed, and Parmesan cheese on top.

Nutrition:

- Calories: 230
- Fat: 10 g
- Protein: 8 g
- Sugar: 5 g

34.   Braised Fennel

Preparation Time: 10−20 minutes

Cooking Time: 14 minutes

Servings: 4

Ingredients:

- 2 fennel bulbs, trimmed and cut into quarters
- 3 tbsp. extra-virgin olive oil
- 1/4 cup white wine
- 1/4 cup Parmesan, grated
- 3/4 cup veggie stock

- 1/2 lemon juice
- 1 garlic clove; chopped.
- 1 dried red pepper
- Salt and black pepper to the taste

Directions:

1. Set your air fryer oven on "Sauté" mode; add oil and heat it.
2. Add garlic and red pepper, then stir well. Cook for 2 minutes and discard garlic.
3. Add fennel, stir and brown it for 8 minutes.
4. Add salt, pepper, stock, wine, close the lid and cook at high for 4 minutes.
5. Quickly release the pressure, open the air fryer oven lid, add lemon juice, more salt and pepper if needed, and cheese.
6. Mix to coat, divide among plates and serve.

Nutrition:

- Calories: 230
- Fat: 4 g
- Protein: 1 g
- Sugar: 3 g

35.   Brussels Sprouts & Potatoes Dish

Preparation Time: 10−20 minutes

Cooking Time: 5 minutes

Servings: 4

Ingredients:

- 1 ½ lb. brussels sprouts, washed and trimmed
- 1 ½ tbsp. breadcrumbs
- 1/2 cup beef stock
- 1 cup new potatoes, chopped
- 1 ½ tbsp. butter
- Salt and black pepper to taste

Directions:

1. Put sprouts and potatoes in your air fryer oven.
2. Add stock, salt, and pepper, close the lid and cook at high for 5 minutes.
3. Quickly release the pressure, open the lid; set on "Sauté" mode; add butter and breadcrumbs, toss to coat well, divide among plates and serve.

Nutrition:

- Calories: 150
- Fat: 8 g
- Protein: 1 g
- Sugar: 2 g

36.   Beet and Orange Salad

Preparation Time: 10−20 minutes

Cooking Time: 7 minutes

Servings: 4

Ingredients:

- 1 ½ lb. beets
- 3 strips orange peel
- 2 tbsp. cider vinegar
- 1/2 cup orange juice
- 2 tsp. orange zest, grated
- 2 tbsp. brown sugar
- 2 scallions, chopped
- 2 tsp. mustard
- 2 cups arugula and mustard greens

Directions:

1. Scrub beets well cut them in halves, and put them in a bowl.
2. In your air fryer oven, mix orange peel strips with vinegar and orange juice and stir.
3. Add beets, seal the air fryer oven lid, cook at high for 7 minutes, and naturally release the pressure.
4. Carefully open the lid, take beets and transfer them to a bowl.
5. Discard peel strips from the pot, add mustard and sugar, and stir well.
6. Add scallions, grated orange zest to beets, and toss them.
7. Add liquid from the pot over beets, toss to coat and serve on plates on top of mixed salad greens.

Nutrition:

- Calories: 164

- Fat: 5 g
- Protein: 2 g
- Sugar: 5 g

37.   Endives Dish

Preparation Time: 10−20 minutes

Cooking Time: 7 minutes

Servings: 4

Ingredients:

- 4 endives, trimmed
- 2 tbsp. butter
- 1 tbsp. white flour
- 4 slices ham
- 1/2 tsp. nutmeg
- 14 oz. milk
- Salt and black pepper to taste

Directions:

1. Put the endives in the steamer basket of your air fryer oven, add some water to the pot, cover, and cook at high for 10 minutes.
2. Meanwhile, heat a pan with the butter over medium heat, stir and melt it.
3. Add flour, stir well and cook for 3 minutes.
4. Add milk, salt, pepper, and nutmeg, stir well, reduce heat to low, and cook for 10 minutes.
5. Release the pressure from the pot, uncover it, transfer them to a cutting board and roll each in a slice of ham.

6. Arrange endives in a pan, add the milk mixture over them, introduce in preheated broiler and cook for 10 minutes. Slice, arrange on plates and serve.

Nutrition:

- Calories: 175
- Fat: 8 g
- Protein: 1 g
- Sugar: 2 g

38. Roasted Potatoes

Preparation Time: 10–20 minutes

Cooking Time: 17 minutes

Servings: 4

Ingredients:

- 2 lb. baby potatoes
- 5 tbsp. vegetable oil
- 1/2 cup stock
- 1 rosemary spring
- 5 garlic cloves
- Salt and black pepper to taste

Directions:

1. Set your air fryer oven on "Sauté" mode; add oil and heat it.
2. Add potatoes, rosemary and garlic, stir and brown them for 10 minutes.

3. Prick each potato with a knife, add the stock, salt, and pepper to the pot, seal the air fryer oven lid and cook at high for 7 minutes.
4. Quickly release the pressure, open the air fryer oven lid, divide potatoes among plates and serve.

Nutrition:

- Calories: 250
- Fat: 15 g
- Protein: 2 g
- Sugar: 1 g

39. Cabbage Wedges

Preparation Time: 10 minutes

Cooking Time: 29 minutes

Servings: 2

Ingredients:

- 1 small head green cabbage
- 6 strips bacon, thick-cut, pastured
- 1 tsp. onion powder
- 1/2 tsp. ground black pepper
- 1 tsp. garlic powder
- 3/4 tsp. salt
- 1/4 tsp. red chili flakes
- 1/2 tsp. fennel seeds
- 3 tbsp. olive oil

Directions:

1. Switch on the air fryer, insert fryer basket, grease it with olive oil, then shut with its lid, set the fryer to 350°F, and preheat for 5 minutes.

2. Open the fryer, add bacon strips in it, close with its lid and cook for 10 minutes until nicely golden and crispy, turning the bacon halfway through the frying.

3. Meanwhile, prepare the cabbage, remove the cabbage's outer leaves, and then cut it into 8 wedges, keeping the core intact.

4. Prepare the spice mix and for this, place onion powder in a bowl, add black pepper, garlic powder, salt, red chili, and fennel and stir until mixed.

5. Drizzle cabbage wedges with oil and then sprinkle with spice mix until well coated.

6. When the air fryer beeps, open its lid, transfer bacon strips to a cutting board and let it rest.

7. Add seasoned cabbage wedges into the fryer basket, close with its lid, then cook for 8 minutes at 400°F, flip the cabbage, spray with oil and continue air frying for 6 minutes until nicely golden and cooked.

8. When done, transfer cabbage wedges to a plate.

9. Chop the bacon, sprinkle it over cabbage and serve.

Nutrition:

- Calories: 123
- Carbs: 2 g
- Fat: 11 g
- Protein: 4 g
- Fiber: 0 g
- Sugar: 1 g

40. Creamed Spinach

Preparation Time: 10 minutes

Cooking Time: 20 minutes

Servings: 2

Ingredients:

- 1/2 cup chopped white onion
- 10 oz. frozen spinach, thawed
- 1 tsp. salt
- 1 tsp. ground black pepper
- 2 tsp. minced garlic
- 1/2 tsp. ground nutmeg
- 4 oz. cream cheese, reduced-fat, diced
- 1/4 cup shredded Parmesan cheese, reduced-fat
- 2 tbsp of olive oil

Directions:

1. Switch on the air fryer, insert fryer basket, grease it with olive oil, then shut with its lid, set the fryer at 350°F, and preheat for 5 minutes.

2. Meanwhile, take a 6-inches baking pan, grease it with oil, and set it aside.

3. Put spinach in a basin, add remaining ingredients except for Parmesan cheese, stir until well mixed and then add the mixture into a prepared baking pan.

4. Open the fryer, add pan in it, close with its lid and cook for 10 minutes until cooked and cheese has melted, stirring halfway through.

5. Then sprinkle Parmesan cheese on top of spinach and continue air frying for 5 minutes at 400°F until the top is nicely golden and cheese has melted.

6. Serve straight away.

Nutrition:

- Calories: 273
- Carbs: 8 g
- Fat: 23 g
- Protein: 8 g
- Fiber: 2 g

41.Eggplant Parmesan

Preparation Time: 20 minutes

Cooking Time: 15 minutes

Servings: 4

Ingredients:

- 1/2 cup and 3 tbsp. almond flour, divided
- 1 ¼ lb. eggplant, ½-inch sliced
- 1 tbsp. chopped parsley
- 1 tsp. Italian seasoning

- 2 tsp. salt
- 1 cup marinara sauce
- 1 egg, pastured
- 1 tbsp. water
- 3 tbsp. grated Parmesan cheese, reduced-fat
- 1/4 cup grated mozzarella cheese, reduced-fat

Directions:

1. Slice the eggplant into ½-inch pieces, place them in a colander, sprinkle with 1 ½ teaspoon of salt on both sides, and let it rest for 15 minutes.

2. Meanwhile, place ½ cup flour in a bowl, add egg and water and whisk until blended.

3. Place remaining flour in a shallow dish, add remaining salt, Italian seasoning, and Parmesan cheese, and stir until mixed.

4. Switch on the air fryer, insert fryer basket, grease it with olive oil, then shut with its lid, set the fryer to 360°F, and preheat for 5 minutes.

5. Meanwhile, drain the eggplant pieces, pat them dry, and then dip each slice into the egg mixture and coat with flour mixture.

6. Open the air fryer, add coated eggplant slices in it in a single layer, close with its lid and cook for 8 minutes until nicely golden and cooked, flipping the eggplant slices halfway through the frying.

7. Then top each eggplant slice with a tbsp. of marinara sauce and some of the Mozzarella

cheese and continue air frying for 1 to 2 minutes or until cheese has melted.

8. When the air fryer beeps, open its lid, transfer eggplants onto a serving plate, and keep them warm.

9. Cook the remaining eggplant slices the same way and serve.

Nutrition:

- Calories: 193
- Carbs: 27 g
- Fat: 5.5 g
- Protein: 10 g
- Fiber: 6 g

CHAPTER 9. LUNCH RECIPES

42. Tilapia with Coconut Rice

Preparation time: 10 minutes

Cooking time: 15 minutes

Servings: 4

Ingredients:

- 4 (6 oz.) boneless tilapia fillets
- 1 tbsp. ground turmeric
- 1 tbsp. olive oil
- 2 (8.8 oz.) packets precooked whole-grain rice
- 1 cup light coconut milk
- 1/2 cup fresh chopped cilantro
- 1 ½ tbsp. fresh lime juice
- Salt and pepper to taste

Directions:

1. Season the fish with turmeric, salt, and pepper.
2. Cook oil in a large skillet at medium heat and add the fish.
3. Cook for 2 to 3 minutes per side until golden brown.
4. Remove the fish to a plate and cover to keep warm.
5. Reheat the skillet and add the rice, coconut milk, and a pinch of salt.
6. Simmer on high heat until thickened, about 3 to 4 minutes.
7. Stir in the cilantro and lime juice.
8. Spoon the rice onto plates and serve with the cooked fish.

Nutrition:

- Calories: 460
- Carbohydrates: 27.1 g
- Fiber: 3.7 g

43. Spicy Turkey Tacos

Preparation time: 5 minutes

Cooking time: 25 minutes

Servings: 2

Ingredients:

- 1 tbsp. olive oil
- 1 medium yellow onion, diced
- 2 cloves minced garlic
- 1 lb. 93% lean ground turkey
- 1 cup tomato sauce, no sugar added
- 1 jalapeno, seeded and minced
- 8 low-carb multigrain tortillas
- 1 tbsp. taco seasoning
- 1 tbsp. cayenne

Directions:

1. Heat up oil in a big skillet over medium heat.
2. Add the onion and sauté for 4 minutes then stir in the garlic and cook 1 minute more.
3. Stir in the ground turkey and cook for 5 minutes until browned, breaking it up with a wooden spoon.
4. Sprinkle on the taco seasoning and cayenne then stir well.
5. Cook for 30 seconds and mix in the tomato sauce and jalapeno.
6. Simmer on low heat for 10 minutes while you warm the tortillas in the microwave.
7. Serve the meat in the tortillas with your favorite taco toppings.

Nutrition:

- Calories: 195
- Carbohydrates: 15.4 g
- Fiber: 8 g

44.   Quick and Easy Shrimp Stir-Fry

Preparation time: 15 minutes

Cooking time: 15 minutes

Servings: 2

Ingredients:

- 1 tbsp. olive oil
- 1 lb. uncooked shrimp
- 1 tbsp. sesame oil
- 8 oz. snow peas
- 4 oz. broccoli, chopped
- 1 medium red pepper, sliced
- 3 cloves minced garlic
- 1 tbsp. fresh grated ginger
- 1/2 cup soy sauce
- 1 tbsp. cornstarch
- 2 tbsp. fresh lime juice
- 1/4 tsp. liquid Stevia extract

Directions:

1. Cook olive oil in a huge skillet over medium heat.
2. Add the shrimp and season then sauté for 5 minutes.
3. Remove the shrimp to a bowl and keep warm.
4. Reheat the skillet with the sesame oil and add the veggies.
5. Sauté until the veggies are tender, about 6 to 8 minutes.
6. Cook garlic and ginger for 1 minute more.
7. Whisk together the remaining ingredients and pour them into the skillet.
8. Toss to coat the veggies then add the shrimp and reheat.

Nutrition:

- Calories: 220
- Carbohydrates: 12.7 g
- Fiber: 2.6 g

45. Chicken Burrito Bowl with Quinoa

Preparation time: 15 minutes

Cooking time: 10 minutes

Servings: 2

Ingredients:

- 1 tbsp. chipotle chills in adobo
- 1 tbsp. olive oil
- 1/2 tsp. garlic powder
- 1/2 tsp. ground cumin
- 1 lb. boneless skinless chicken breast
- 2 cups cooked quinoa
- 2 cups shredded romaine lettuce
- 1 cup black beans
- 1 cup diced avocado
- 3 tbsp. fat-free sour cream
- Salt and pepper to taste

Directions:

1. Stir together the chipotle chills, olive oil, garlic powder, and cumin in a small bowl.

2. Preheat a grill pan to medium-high and grease with cooking spray.

3. Season the chicken with salt and pepper and add to the grill pan.

4. Grill for 5 minutes then flip it and brush with the chipotle glaze.

5. Cook for another 3 to 5 minutes until cooked through.

6. Remove to a cutting board and chop the chicken.

7. Assemble the bowls with 1/6 of the quinoa, chicken, lettuce, beans, and avocado.

8. Top each with a half tbsp. of fat-free sour cream to serve.

Nutrition:

- Calories: 410
- Carbohydrates: 37.4 g
- Fiber: 8.5 g

46. Baked Salmon Cakes

Preparation time: 10 minutes

Cooking time: 20 minutes

Servings: 4

Ingredients:

- 15 oz. canned salmon, drained

- 1 large egg, whisked
- 2 tsp. Dijon mustard
- 1 small yellow onion, minced
- 1 1/2 cups whole-wheat breadcrumbs
- 1/4 cup low-fat mayonnaise
- 1/4 cup nonfat Greek yogurt, plain
- 1 tbsp. fresh chopped parsley
- 1 tbsp. fresh lemon juice
- 2 green onions, sliced thin

Directions:

1. Set the oven to 450°F and prep the baking sheet with parchment.
2. Flake the salmon into a medium bowl then stir in the egg and mustard.
3. Mix in the onions and breadcrumbs by hand, blending well, then shape into 8 patties.
4. Grease a large skillet and heat it over medium heat.
5. Fry patties for 2 minutes per side.
6. Situate patties to the baking sheet and bake for 15 minutes.
7. Meanwhile, whisk together the remaining ingredients.
8. Serve the Baked Salmon Cakes with creamy herb sauce.

Nutrition:

- Calories: 240
- Carbohydrates: 9.3 g

- Fiber: 1.5 g

47.   Rice and Meatball Stuffed Bell Peppers

Preparation time: 15 minutes

Cooking time: 20 minutes

Servings: 4

Ingredients:

- 4 bell peppers
- 1-tbsp. olive oil
- 1 small onion, chopped
- 2 garlic cloves, minced
- 1 cup frozen cooked rice, thawed
- 16–20 small frozen precooked meatballs
- 1/2 cup tomato sauce
- 2 tbsp. Dijon mustard

Directions:

1. To prepare the peppers, cut off about 1/2-inch of the tops. Carefully take out membranes and seeds from inside the peppers. Set aside.
2. In a 6x6x2-inch pan, combine the olive oil, onion, and garlic. Bake in the air fryer for 2 to 4 minutes or until crisp and tender. Remove the vegetable mixture from the pan and set it aside in a medium bowl.

3. Add the rice, meatballs, tomato sauce, and mustard to the vegetable mixture and stir to combine.
4. Stuff the peppers with the meat-vegetable mixture.
5. Situate peppers in the air fryer basket and bake for 9 to 13 minutes or until the filling is hot and the peppers are tender.

Nutrition:

- Calories: 487
- Carbohydrates: 57 g
- Fiber: 6 g

48.   Stir-Fried Steak and Cabbage

Preparation time: 15 minutes

Cooking time: 10 minutes

Servings: 4

Ingredients:

- 1/2 lb. sirloin steak, cut into strips
- 2 tsp. cornstarch
- 1-tbsp. peanut oil
- 2 cups chopped red or green cabbage
- 1 yellow bell pepper, chopped
- 2 green onions, chopped
- 2 garlic cloves, sliced
- 1/2 cup commercial stir-fry sauce

Directions:

1. Toss the steak with the cornstarch and set aside
2. In a 6-inch metal bowl, combine the peanut oil with the cabbage. Place in the basket and cook for 3 to 4 minutes.
3. Remove the bowl from the basket and add the steak, pepper, onions, and garlic. Return to the air fryer and cook for 3 to 5 minutes.
4. Add the stir-fry sauce and cook for 2 to 4 minutes. Serve over rice.

Nutrition:

- Calories: 180
- Carbohydrates: 9 g
- Fiber: 2 g

49.   Lemon Chicken with Peppers

Preparation time: 5 minutes

Cooking time: 20 minutes

Servings: 3

Ingredients:

- 1 tsp. cornstarch
- 1 tbsp. low sodium soy sauce
- 12 oz. chicken breast tenders, cut in thirds

- 1/4 cup fresh lemon juice
- 1/4 cup low sodium soy sauce
- 1/4 cup fat-free chicken broth
- 1 tsp. fresh ginger, minced
- 2 garlic cloves, minced
- 1 tbsp. Splenda
- 1 tsp. cornstarch
- 1 tbsp. vegetable oil
- 1/4 cup red bell pepper
- 1/4 cup green bell pepper

Directions:

1. Scourge 1 tsp. cornstarch and 1 tbsp. soy sauce. Add sliced chicken tenders. Chill to marinate for 10 minutes.
2. Stir the lemon juice, 1/4 cup soy sauce, chicken broth, ginger, garlic, Splenda, and 1 tsp. cornstarch together.
3. Warm-up oil in a medium frying pan. Cook chicken over medium-high heat for 4 minutes.
4. Add sauce and sliced peppers. Cook 1 to 2 minutes more.

Nutrition:

- Calories: 150
- Carbohydrates: 6 g
- Fiber: 1 g

50.   Dijon Herb Chicken

Preparation time: 7 minutes

Cooking time: 25 minutes

Servings: 4

Ingredients:

- 4 skinless, boneless chicken breast halves
- 1 tbsp. butter
- 1 tbsp. olive or vegetable oil
- 2 garlic cloves, finely minced
- 1/2 cup dry white wine
- 1/4 cup water
- 2 tbsp. Dijon-style mustard
- 1/2 tsp. dried dill weed
- 1/4 tsp. coarsely ground pepper
- 1/3 cups chopped fresh parsley
- Salt to taste

Directions:

1. Situate chicken breasts between sheets of plastic wrap or waxed paper, and lb. with a kitchen mallet until they are evenly about 1/4-inch thick.
2. Warm-up butter and oil over medium-high heat; cook chicken pieces for 3 minutes per side. Transfer chicken to a platter; keep warm and set aside.

3. Sauté garlic for 15 seconds in skillet drippings; stir in wine, water, mustard, dill weed, salt, and pepper. Boil and reduce volume by 1/2, stirring up the browned bits at the bottom of the skillet.

4. Drizzle sauce over chicken cutlets. Sprinkle with parsley and serve.

Nutrition:

- Calories: 223
- Carbohydrates: 6 g
- Fiber: 1 g

51. Sesame Chicken Stir Fry

Preparation time: 10 minutes

Cooking time: 30 minutes

Servings: 2

Ingredients:

- 12 oz. skinless, boneless chicken breast
- 1 tbsp. vegetable oil
- 2 garlic cloves, finely minced
- 1 cup broccoli florets
- 1 cup cauliflowers
- 1/2 lb. fresh mushrooms, sliced
- 4 green onions, cut into 1-inch pieces
- 2 tbsp. low-sodium soy sauce
- 3 tbsp. dry sherry

- 1 tsp. finely minced fresh ginger
- 1/4 tsp. sesame oil
- 1/4 cup dry-roasted peanuts
- ¼ cup arrowroot

Directions:

1. Cut off fat from chicken and thinly slice diagonally into 1-inch strips.

2. In a huge non-stick skillet, heat oil and stir-fry chicken for 4 minutes Remove; put aside and keep warm.

3. Stir-fry garlic for 15 seconds; then broccoli and cauliflower, stir-fry for 2 minutes. Then fry mushrooms, green onions, soy sauce, sherry, and ginger for 2 minutes.

4. Pour dissolved arrowroot, sesame oil, peanuts, and chicken. Cook until heated through and the sauce has thickened.

Nutrition:

- Calories: 256
- Carbohydrates: 9 g
- Protein: 30 g

52. Rosemary Chicken

Preparation time: 9 minutes

Cooking time: 30 minutes

Servings: 4

Ingredients:

- 1 (2 1/2–3 lb.) broiler-fryer chicken
- Salt and ground black pepper to taste
- 4 garlic cloves, finely minced
- 1 tsp. dried rosemary
- 1/4 cup dry white wine
- 1/4 cup chicken broth

Directions:

1. Preheat broiler.
2. Season chicken with salt and pepper. Place in broiler pan. Broil 5 minutes per side.
3. Situate chicken, garlic, rosemary, wine, and broth in a Dutch oven. Cook, covered, at medium heat for about 30 minutes, turning once.

Nutrition:

- Calories: 176
- Carbohydrates: 1 g
- Fat: 1 g

53. Pepper Chicken Skillet

Preparation time: 10 minutes

Cooking time: 35 minutes

Servings: 4

Ingredients:

- 1 tbsp. vegetable oil

- 12 oz. skinless, boneless chicken breasts
- 2 garlic cloves, finely minced
- 3 bell peppers (red green and yellow)
- 2 medium onions, sliced
- 1 tsp. ground cumin
- 1 1/2 tsp. dried oregano leaves
- 2 tsp. chopped fresh jalapeño peppers
- 3 tbsp. fresh lemon juice
- 2 tbsp. chopped fresh parsley
- 1/4 tsp. salt
- Pepper to taste

Directions:

1. In a big non-stick skillet, heat oil at medium-high heat; stir-fry chicken for 4 minutes.
2. Cook garlic for 15 seconds, stirring constantly. Fry bell pepper strips, sliced onion, cumin, oregano, and chilies for 2 to 3 minutes.
3. Toss lemon juice, parsley, salt, and pepper and serve.

Nutrition:

- Calories: 174
- Carbohydrate: 6 g
- Protein: 21 g

54.   Dijon Salmon

Preparation time: 8 minutes

Cooking time: 26 minutes

Servings: 3

Ingredients:

- 1 tbsp. olive oil
- 1 1/2 lb. salmon fillets, cut into 6 pieces
- 1/4 cup lemon juice
- 2 tbsp. Equal (sugar substitute)
- 2 tbsp. Dijon mustard
- 1 tbsp. stick butter or margarine
- 1 tbsp. capers
- 1 garlic clove, minced
- 2 tbsp. chopped fresh dill

Directions:

1. Heat up olive oil in a huge non-stick skillet over medium heat. Add salmon and cook for 5 minutes, turning once. Reduce heat to medium-low; cover. Cook 6 to 8 minutes or until salmon flakes easily with a fork.
2. Remove salmon from skillet to serving plate; keep warm.
3. Add lemon juice, Equal, mustard, butter, capers, and garlic to the skillet. Cook at medium heat for 3 minutes, stirring frequently.
4. To serve, spoon sauce over salmon. Sprinkle with dill.

Nutrition:

- Calories: 252
- Carbohydrates: 2 g
- Protein: 23 g

55.   Pulled Pork

Preparation time: 10 minutes

Cooking time: 35 minutes

Servings: 3

Ingredients:

- 1 whole pork tenderloin
- 1 tsp. chili powder
- 1/2 tsp. garlic powder
- 1/2 cup onion
- 1 1/2 tsp. garlic
- 1 (14.5 oz.) can of tomatoes
- 1 tbsp. cider vinegar
- 1 tbsp. prepared mustard
- 1–2 tsp. chili powder
- 1/4 tsp. maple extract
- 1/4 tsp. liquid smoke
- 1/3 cup Equal (sugar substitute)
- 6 multigrain hamburger buns
- Cooking spray

Directions:

1. Season pork with 1 tsp. chili powder and garlic powder; situate in baking pan. Bake in preheated 220°C ovens for 30 to 40 minutes. Set aside for 15 minutes. Slice into 2 to 3-inch slices; shred slices into bite-size pieces with a fork.

2. Coat medium saucepan with cooking spray. Cook onion and garlic for 5 minutes. Cook tomatoes, vinegar, mustard, chili powder, maple extract, and liquid smoke to the saucepan. Allow to boil; decrease heat.

3. Simmer, uncovered, 10 to 15 minutes. Sprinkle Equal

4. Stir in pork into sauce. Cook 2 to 3 minutes. Spoon mixture into buns.

Nutrition:

- Calories: 252
- Carbohydrates: 29 g
- Protein: 21 g

56. Herb Lemon Salmon

Preparation time: 10 minutes

Cooking time: 27 minutes

Servings: 2

Ingredients:

- 2 cups water
- 2/3 cup Farro
- 1 medium eggplant
- 1 red bell pepper
- 1 summer squash
- 1 small onion
- 1 1/2 cups cherry tomatoes
- 3 tbsp. extra-virgin olive oil
- 3/4 tsp. salt, divided
- 1/2 tsp. ground pepper
- 2 tbsp. capers
- 1 tbsp. red-wine vinegar
- 2 tsp. honey
- 1 1/4 lb. salmon cut into 4 portions
- 1 tsp. lemon zest
- 1/2 tsp. Italian seasoning
- Lemon wedges for serving
- Cooking spray

Directions:

1. Situate racks in upper and lower thirds of the oven; set to 450°F. Prep 2 rimmed baking sheets with foil and coat with cooking spray.

2. Boil water and Farro. Adjust heat to low, cover, and simmer for 30 minutes. Drain if necessary.

3. Mix eggplant, bell pepper, squash, onion, and tomatoes with oil, 1/2 tsp. salt, and 1/4 tsp. pepper. Portion between the baking sheets. Roast on the upper and

lower racks, stir once halfway, for 25 minutes. Put them back to the bowl. Mix in capers, vinegar, and honey.

4. Rub salmon with lemon zest, Italian seasoning, and the remaining 1/4 tsp. each salt and pepper and situate on one of the baking sheets.

5. Roast on the lower rack for 12 minutes, depending on thickness. Serve with Farro, vegetable caponata, and lemon wedges.

Nutrition:

- Calories: 450
- Carbohydrates: 41 g
- Fat: 17 g

57. Ginger Chicken

Preparation time: 10 minutes

Cooking time: 25 minutes

Servings: 4

Ingredients:

- 2 tbsp. vegetable oil, divided use
- 1 lb. boneless, skinless chicken breasts
- 1 cup red bell pepper strips
- 1 cup sliced fresh mushrooms
- 16 fresh pea pods, cut in half crosswise
- 1/2 cup sliced water chestnuts
- 1/4 cup sliced green onions
- 1 tbsp. grated fresh ginger root
- 1 large garlic clove, crushed
- 2/3 cup reduced-fat, reduced-sodium chicken broth
- 2 tbsp. Equal (sugar substitute)
- 2 tbsp. light soy sauce
- 4 tsp. cornstarch
- 2 tsp. dark sesame oil

Directions:

1. Heat up 1 tbsp. vegetable oil in a huge skillet over medium-high heat. Stir fry chicken until no longer pink. Remove chicken from skillet.

2. Heat the remaining 1 tbsp. vegetable oil in a skillet. Add red peppers, mushrooms, pea pods, water chestnuts, green onion, ginger, and garlic. Stir fry mixture for 3 to 4 minutes until vegetables are crisp-tender.

3. Meanwhile, combine chicken broth, Equal, soy sauce, cornstarch, and sesame oil until smooth. Stir into skillet mixture. Cook at medium heat until thick and clear. Stir in chicken; heat through. Season with salt and pepper to taste, if desired.

4. Serve over hot cooked rice, if desired.

Nutrition:

- Calories: 263
- Carbohydrates: 11 g
- Fat: 11 g

58.   Teriyaki Chicken

Preparation time: 7 minutes

Cooking time: 26 minutes

Servings: 4

Ingredients:

- 1 tbsp. cornstarch
- 1 tbsp. cold water
- 1/2 cup Splenda
- 1/2 cup soy sauce
- 1/4 cup cider vinegar
- 1 garlic clove, minced
- 1/2 tsp. ground ginger
- 1/4 tsp. ground black pepper
- 12 skinless, boneless chicken breast halves

Directions:

1. In a small saucepan in low heat, mix cornstarch, cold water, Splenda, soy sauce, vinegar, garlic, ginger, and ground black pepper. Let simmer, stirring frequently, until sauce thickens and bubbles.
2. Preheat oven to 425°F (220°C).
3. Position chicken pieces in a lightly greased 9x13-inch baking dish. Brush chicken with the sauce. Turn pieces over, and brush again.
4. Bake in the prepared oven for 30 minutes. Turn pieces over, and bake for another 30 minutes. Brush with sauce every 10 minutes during cooking.

Nutrition:

- Calories: 140
- Carbohydrates: 3 g
- Protein: 25 g

59.   Roasted Garlic Salmon

Preparation time: 8 minutes

Cooking time: 45 minutes

Servings: 2

Ingredients:

- 14 large garlic cloves
- 1/4 cup olive oil
- 2 tbsp. fresh oregano
- 1 tsp. salt
- 3/4 tsp. pepper
- 6 cups Brussels sprouts
- 3/4 cup white wine, preferably Chardonnay
- 2 lb. wild-caught salmon fillet

Directions:

1. Prep oven at 450°F.
2. Finely chopped 2 garlic cloves and combine in a small bowl with oil, 1 tbsp. oregano, 1/2 tsp. salt, and 1/4 tsp. pepper. Slice remaining garlic and mix in Brussels sprouts and 3 tbsp. the seasoned oil in a big roasting pan. Roast, stirring once, for 15 minutes.
3. Pour in wine into the remaining oil mixture. Remove from oven, stir the vegetables and situate salmon on top. Dash with the wine mixture. Sprinkle with the remaining 1 tbsp. oregano and 1/2 tsp. each salt and pepper.
4. Bake for 10 minutes more. Serve with lemon wedges.

Nutrition:

- Calories: 334
- Carbohydrates: 10 g
- Protein: 33 g

60. Lemon Sesame Halibut

Preparation time: 9 minutes

Cooking time: 29 minutes

Servings: 4

Ingredients:

- 2 tbsp. lemon juice
- 2 tbsp. extra-virgin olive oil
- 1 garlic clove, minced
- Freshly ground pepper, to taste
- 2 tbsp. sesame seeds
- 1 1/2 lb. halibut, or mahi-mahi, cut into 4 portions
- 1 1/2–2 tsp. dried thyme leaves
- 1/4 tsp. coarse sea salt, or kosher salt
- Lemon wedges

Directions:

1. Preheat oven to 450°F. Line a baking sheet with foil.
2. Place lemon juice, oil, garlic, and pepper in a shallow glass dish. Add fish and turn to coat. Wrap and marinate for 15 minutes.
3. Fry sesame seeds in a small dry skillet over medium-low heat, stirring constantly, for 3 minutes. Set aside to cool. Mix in thyme.
4. Season the fish with salt and coat evenly with the sesame seed mixture, covering the sides as well as the top. Transfer the fish to the prepared baking sheet and roast until just opaque in the center, 10 to 14 minutes. Serve with lemon wedges.

Nutrition:

- Calories: 225
- Carbohydrates: 2 g
- Fat: 11 g

61. Turkey Sausage Casserole

Preparation time: 12 minutes

Cooking time: 32 minutes

Servings: 4

Ingredients:

- 5 oz. turkey breakfast sausage, casings removed
- 1 tsp. canola oil
- 1 onion, chopped
- 1 red bell pepper, chopped
- 4 large eggs
- 4 large egg whites
- 2 1/2 cups low-fat milk
- 1 tsp. dry mustard
- 1/2 tsp. salt
- 1/4 tsp. freshly ground pepper
- 2/3 cup low-fat Cheddar cheese, divided
- 10 slices white bread, crusts removed
- Cooking spray

Directions:

1. Grease a 9x13-inch baking dish with cooking spray.
2. Fry sausage in a skillet over medium heat, crumbling with a fork until browned. Transfer to a bowl.
3. Cook oil, onion, and bell pepper to skillet; stirring occasionally, for 5 minutes. Fry sausage for 5 minutes more. Remove from heat and set aside.
4. Scourge eggs and egg whites in a large bowl until blended. Whisk in milk, mustard, salt, and pepper. Stir in 1/3 cup cheddar.
5. Arrange bread in a single layer in a prepared baking dish. Pour egg mixture over bread and top with reserved vegetables and sausage. Sprinkle with remaining 1/3 cup Cheddar. Seal with plastic wrap and chill for at least 5 hours or overnight.
6. Preheat oven to 350°F. Bake casserole, uncovered, until set and puffed 40 to 50 minutes.

Nutrition:

- Calories: 141
- Carbohydrates: 10 g
- Protein: 10 g

CHAPTER 10. FISH & SEAFOOD LUNCH RECIPES

64.   Salmon Cakes in Air Fryer

Preparation Time: 9 minutes

Cooking Time: 7 minutes

Servings: 2

Ingredients:

- 8 oz. fresh salmon fillet
- 1 egg
- 1/8 salt
- 1/4 garlic powder
- 1 Sliced lemon

Directions:

1. In the bowl, chop the salmon, add the egg and spices.
2. Form tiny cakes.
3. Let the air fryer preheat to 390°F. On the bottom of the air fryer bowl lay sliced lemons—place cakes on top.
4. Cook them for 7 minutes. Based on your diet preferences, eat with your chosen dip.

Nutrition:

- Calories: 194
- Fat: 9 g
- Carbs: 1 g
- Proteins: 25 g

65.   Coconut Shrimp

Preparation Time: 9 minutes

Cooking Time: 8-10 minutes

Servings: 4

Ingredients:

- 1/2 cup pork rinds: ½ cup (Crushed)
- 4 cups jumbo shrimp: 4 cups. (deveined)
- 1/2 cup coconut flakes, preferably
- 2 eggs
- 1/2 cup coconut flour
- 1/2 inch any your choice oil for frying
- Freshly ground black pepper and kosher salt to taste

Dipping sauce:

- 2-3 tbsp. powdered sugar as a substitute
- 3 tbsp. mayonnaise
- 1/2 cup sour cream
- 1/4 tsp. coconut extract or to taste
- 3 tbsp. coconut cream
- 1/4 tsp. pineapple flavoring as much to taste.
- 3 tbsp. coconut flakes preferably unsweetened (optional)

Directions:

Sauce:

1. Mix all the ingredients into a tiny bowl for the dipping sauce (Pineapple flavor). Combine well and put in the fridge until ready to serve.

Shrimps:

1. Whip all eggs in a deep bowl and in a small shallow bowl; add the crushed pork rinds, coconut flour, sea salt, coconut flakes, and freshly ground black pepper.
2. Put the shrimp one by one in the mixed eggs for dipping, then in the coconut flour blend. Put them on a clean plate or put them on your air fryer's basket.
3. Place the shrimp battered in a single layer on your air fryer basket. Spritz the shrimp with oil and cook for 8 to 10 minutes at 360°F, flipping them through halfway.
4. Enjoy hot with dipping sauce.

Nutrition:

- Calories: 340
- Proteins: 25 g
- Carbs: 9 g
- Fat: 16 g

66. Crispy Fish Sticks in Air Fryer

Preparation Time: 9 minutes

Cooking Time: 10 minutes

Servings: 4

Ingredients:

- 1 lb. whitefish such as cod
- 1/4 cup mayonnaise
- 2 tbsp. Dijon mustard
- 2 tbsp. water
- 1 ½ cup pork rind
- 3/4 tsp. Cajun seasoning
- Kosher salt and pepper to taste
- Cooking spray

Directions:

1. Spray with non-stick cooking spray to the air fryer rack.
2. Pat the fish dry and cut into sticks about 1 inch by 2 inches' broad
3. Stir together the mayonnaise, mustard, and water in a tiny small dish. Mix the pork rinds and Cajun seasoning into another small container.
4. Adding kosher salt and pepper to taste (both pork rinds and seasoning can have a decent amount of kosher salt, so you can dip a finger to see how salty it is).
5. Working for one slice of fish at a time, dip to cover in the mayonnaise mix, and then tap off the excess. Dip into the mixture of pork rind, then flip to cover. Place on the rack of an air fryer.

6. Set at 400°F to air fry for 5 minutes, then turn the fish with tongs and bake for another 5 minutes. Serve.

Nutrition:

- Calories: 263
- Fat: 16 g
- Carbs: 1 g
- Proteins: 26.4 g

67. Honey-Glazed Salmon

Preparation Time: 11 minutes

Cooking Time: 16 minutes

Servings: 2

Ingredients:

- 6 tsp. gluten-free soy sauce
- 2 pcs. Salmon fillets
- 3 tsp. sweet rice wine
- 1 tsp. water
- 6 tbsp. honey

Directions:

1. In a bowl, mix sweet rice wine, soy sauce, honey, and water.
2. Set half of it aside.
3. In half of it, marinate the fish and let it rest for 2 hours.
4. Let the air fryer preheat to 180°C.

5. Cook the fish for 8 minutes, flip halfway through, and cook for another 5 minutes.
6. Baste the salmon with marinade mixture after 3 or 4 minutes.
7. The half of marinade, pour in a saucepan, reduce to half, serve with a sauce.

Nutrition:

- Calories: 254
- Fat: 12 g
- Carbs: 9.9 g
- Proteins: 20 g

68. Basil-Parmesan Crusted Salmon

Preparation Time: 5 minutes

Cooking Time: 7 minutes

Servings: 4

Ingredients:

- 3 tbsp. grated Parmesan
- 4 skinless salmon fillets
- 1/4 tsp. salt
- Freshly ground black pepper
- 3 tbsp. low-fat mayonnaise
- ¼ cup basil leaves, chopped
- 1/2 lemon
- Olive oil for spraying

Directions:

1. Let the air fryer preheat to 400°F. Spray the basket with olive oil.
2. With salt, pepper, and lemon juice, season the salmon.
3. In a bowl, mix 2 tablespoons of Parmesan cheese with mayonnaise and basil leaves.
4. Add this mix and more parmesan on top of salmon and cook for 7 minutes or until fully cooked.
5. Serve hot.

Nutrition:

- Calories: 289
- Fat: 18.5 g
- Carbs: 1.5 g
- Proteins: 30 g

69.   Cajun Shrimp in Air Fryer

Preparation Time: 9 minutes

Cooking Time: 3 minutes

Servings: 4

Ingredients:

- 24 extra-jumbo shrimp, peeled,
- 2 tbsp. olive oil
- 1 tbsp. Cajun seasoning
- 1 zucchini, thick slices (half-moons)
- 1/4 cup cooked turkey

- 2 yellow squash, sliced half-moons
- 1/4 tsp. kosher salt

Directions:

1. In a bowl, mix the shrimp with Cajun seasoning.
2. In another bowl, add zucchini, turkey, salt, squash, and coat with oil.
3. Let the air fryer preheat to 400°F.
4. Move the shrimp and vegetable mix to the fryer basket and cook for 3 minutes.
5. Serve hot.

Nutrition:

- Calories: 284
- Fat: 14 g
- Carbs: 8 g
- Proteins: 31 g

70.   Crispy Air Fryer Fish

Preparation Time: 11 minutes

Cooking Time: 18 minutes

Servings: 4

Ingredients:

- 2 tsp. old bay
- 4−6, cut in half, whiting fish fillets
- 1/4 cup fine cornmeal
- 1/4 cup flour
- 1 tsp paprika

- 1/2 tsp. garlic powder
- 1 ½ tsp. salt
- ½ freshly ground black pepper

Directions:

1. In a Ziploc bag, add all ingredients and coat the fish fillets with it.
2. Spray oil on the basket of the air fryer and put the fish in it.
3. Cook for ten minutes at 400°F. Flip fish if necessary and coat with oil spray and cook for another 7 minutes.
4. Serve with salad green.

Nutrition:

- Calories: 254
- Fat: 12.7 g
- Carbs: 8.2 g
- Proteins: 17.5 g

71. Air Fryer Lemon Cod

Preparation Time: 5 minutes

Cooking Time: 10 minutes

Servings: 1

Ingredients:

- 1 cod fillet
- 1 tbsp. chopped dried parsley
- Kosher salt and pepper to taste
- 1 tbsp. garlic powder

- 1 lemon

Directions:

1. In a bowl, mix all ingredients and coat the fish fillet with spices.
2. Slice the lemon and lay it at the bottom of the air fryer basket.
3. Put spiced fish on top. Cover the fish with lemon slices.
4. Cook for 10 minutes at 375°F, the internal temperature of fish should be 145°F.
5. Serve.

Nutrition:

- Calories: 101
- Fat: 1 g
- Carbs: 10 g
- Proteins: 16g

72. Air Fryer Salmon Fillets

Preparation Time: 5 minutes

Cooking Time: 15 minutes

Servings: 2

Ingredients:

- 1/4 cup low-fat Greek yogurt
- 2 salmon fillets
- 1 tbsp. fresh dill (chopped)
- 1 lemon juice
- 1/2 garlic powder

- Kosher salt and pepper

Directions:

1. Cut the lemon into slices and lay it at the bottom of the air fryer basket.
2. Season the salmon with kosher salt and pepper. Put salmon on top of lemons.
3. Let it cook at 330°F for 15 minutes.
4. In the meantime, mix garlic powder, lemon juice, salt, pepper with yogurt and dill.
5. Serve the fish with sauce.

Nutrition:

- Calories: 194
- Fat: 7 g
- Carbs: 6 g
- Proteins: 25 g

73.   Air Fryer Fish and Chips

Preparation Time: 11 minutes

Cooking Time: 35 minutes

Servings: 4

Ingredients:

- 4 cups any fish fillet
- 1/4 cup flour
- 1 cup whole-wheat breadcrumbs
- 1 egg
- 2 tbsp. oil
- 2 potatoes

- 1 tsp. salt

Directions:

1. Cut the potatoes in fries. Then coat with oil and salt.
2. Cook in the air fryer for 20 minutes at 400°F, toss the fries halfway through.
3. In the meantime, coat fish in flour, then in the whisked egg, and finally in breadcrumbs mix.
4. Place the fish in the air fryer and let it cook at 330°F for 15 minutes.
5. Flip it halfway through, if needed.
6. Serve with tartar sauce and salad green.

Nutrition:

- Calories: 409
- Fat: 11 g
- Carbs: 44 g
- Proteins: 30 g

74.   Grilled Salmon with Lemon

Preparation Time: 9 minutes

Cooking Time: 8 minutes

Servings: 4

Ingredients:

- 2 tbsp. olive oil
- 2 salmon fillets

- 1/3 cup lemon juice
- 1/3 cup water
- 1/3 cup gluten-free light soy sauce
- 1/3 cup honey
- Scallion slices to garnish
- Freshly ground black pepper, garlic powder, kosher salt to taste

Directions:

1. Season salmon with pepper and salt.
2. In a bowl, mix honey, soy sauce, lemon juice, water, oil. Add salmon to this marinade and let it rest for at least 2 hours.
3. Let the air fryer preheat at 180°C.
4. Place fish in the air fryer and cook for 8 minutes.
5. Move to a dish and top with scallion slices.

Nutrition:

- Calories: 211
- Fat: 9 g
- Carbs: 4.9 g
- Proteins: 15 g

75.   Air-Fried Fish Nuggets

Preparation Time: 15 minutes

Cooking Time: 12 minutes

Servings: 4

Ingredients:

- 2 cups (skinless) fish fillets in cubes
- 1 egg beaten
- 5 tbsp. flour
- 5 tbsp. water
- Kosher salt and pepper to taste
- ½ cup breadcrumbs mix
- 1/4 cup whole-wheat breadcrumbs
- Oil for spraying

Directions:

1. Season the fish cubes with kosher salt and pepper.
2. In a bowl, add flour and gradually add water, mixing as you add.
3. Then mix in the egg. And keep mixing but do not over mix.
4. Coat the cubes in batter, then in the breadcrumb mix. Coat well.
5. Place the cubes in a baking tray and spray with oil.
6. Let the air fryer preheat to 200°C.
7. Place cubes in the air fryer and cook for 12 minutes or until well cooked and golden brown.
8. Serve with salad greens.

Nutrition:

- Calories: 184
- Fat: 3 g
- Carbs: 10 g
- Proteins: 19 g

76. Garlic Rosemary Grilled Prawns

Preparation Time: 5 minutes

Cooking Time: 11 minutes

Servings: 2

Ingredients:

- 1/2 tbsp. melted butter
- 8 green capsicum slices
- 8 prawns
- 1/8 cup rosemary leaves
- Kosher salt and freshly ground black pepper
- 3-4 cloves minced garlic

Directions:

1. In a bowl, mix all the ingredients and marinate the prawns in it for at least 60 minutes or more.
2. Add 2 prawns and 2 slices of capsicum on each skewer.
3. Let the air fryer preheat to 180°C.
4. Cook for 5 to 6 minutes. Then change the temperature to 200°C and cook for another 5 minutes.
5. Serve with lemon wedges.

Nutrition:

- Calories: 194
- Fat: 10 g
- Carbs: 12 g
- Proteins: 26 g

CHAPTER 11. LUNCH LAMB RECIPES

77. Greek Lamb Pita Pockets

Preparation Time: 15 minutes

Cooking Time: 5–7 minutes

Servings: 4

Ingredients:

Dressing:

- 1 cup plain Greek yogurt
- 1 tbsp. lemon juice
- 1 tsp. dried dill weed, crushed
- 1 tsp. ground oregano
- 1/2 tsp. salt

Meatballs:

- 1/2-pound (227 g) ground lamb
- 1 tbsp. diced onion
- 1 tsp. dried parsley
- 1 tsp. dried dill weed, crushed
- 1/4 tsp. oregano
- 1/4 tsp. coriander
- 1/4 tsp. ground cumin
- 1/4 tsp. salt
- 4 pita halves

Suggested Toppings:

- Red onion, slivered
- Seedless cucumber, thinly sliced
- Crumbled feta cheese
- Sliced black olives
- Chopped fresh peppers

Directions:

1. Stir dressing ingredients together and refrigerate while preparing lamb.
2. Combine all meatball ingredients in a large bowl and stir to distribute seasonings.
3. Shape meat mixture into 12 small meatballs, rounded or slightly flattened if you prefer.
4. Air fry at 390°F (199°C) for 5 to 7 minutes, until well done. Remove and drain on paper towels.
5. To serve, pile meatballs and your choice of toppings in pita pockets and drizzle with dressing.

Nutrition:

- Calories: 270
- Fat: 14 g
- Protein: 18 g
- Carbs: 18 g
- Fiber: 2 g
- Sugar: 2 g
- Sodium: 618 mg

78.   Rosemary Lamb Chops

Preparation Time: 30 minutes

Cooking Time: 20 minutes

Servings: 2-3

Ingredients:

- 2 tsp. oil
- 1/2 tsp. ground rosemary
- 1/2 tsp. lemon juice
- 1 lb. (454 g) lamb chops, approximately 1-inch thick
- Salt and pepper to taste
- Cooking spray

Directions:

1. Mix the oil, rosemary, and lemon juice and rub into all sides of the lamb chops. Season to taste with salt and pepper.
2. For best flavor, cover lamb chops and allow them to rest in the fridge for 15 to 20 minutes.
3. Spray air fryer basket with non-stick spray and place lamb chops in it.
4. Air fry at 360°F (182°C) for approximately 20 minutes. This will cook chops to medium. The meat will be juicy but have no remaining pink. Air fry for 1 to 2 minutes longer for well-done chops. For rare chops, continue cooking for about 12 minutes and check for doneness.

Nutrition:

- Calories: 237
- Fat: 13 g
- Protein: 30 g
- Carbs: 0 g
- Fiber: 0 g
- Sugar 0 g
- Sodium: 116 mg

79.   Herb Butter Lamb Chops

Preparation Time: 10 minutes

Cooking Time: 5 minutes

Servings: 4

Ingredients:

- 4 lamb chops
- 1 tsp. rosemary, diced
- 1 tbsp. butter
- Pepper
- Salt

Directions:

1. Season lamb chops with pepper and salt.
2. Place the dehydrating tray in a multi-level air fryer basket and insert the basket in the air fryer oven.
3. Place lamb chops on dehydrating tray.

4. Seal pot with air fryer lid and select "Air Fry" mode, then set the temperature to 400°F and timer for 5 minutes.

5. Mix butter and rosemary and spread overcooked lamb chops.

6. Serve and enjoy.

Nutrition:

- Calories: 278
- Fat: 12.8 g
- Carbs: 0.2 g
- Sugar: 0 g
- Protein: 38 g
- Cholesterol: 129 mg

80.   Za'atar Lamb Chops

Preparation Time: 10 minutes

Cooking Time: 10 minutes

Servings: 4

Ingredients:

- 4 lamb loin chops
- 1/2 tbsp. Za'atar
- 1 tbsp. fresh lemon juice
- 1 tsp. olive oil
- 2 garlic cloves, minced
- Pepper
- Salt

Directions:

1. Coat lamb chops with oil and lemon juice and rubs with Za'atar, garlic, pepper, and salt.

2. Place the dehydrating tray in a multi-level air fryer basket and insert the basket in the air fryer oven.

3. Place lamb chops on dehydrating tray.

4. Seal pot with air fryer lid and select air fry mode, then set the temperature to 400°F and timer for 10 minutes. Turn lamb chops halfway through.

5. Serve and enjoy.

Nutrition:

- Calories: 266
- Fat: 11.2 g
- Carbs: 0.6 g
- Sugar: 0.1 g
- Protein: 38 g
- Cholesterol: 122 mg

81.Greek Lamb Chops

Preparation Time: 10 minutes

Cooking Time: 10 minutes

Servings: 4

Ingredients:

- 2 lb. lamb chops
- 2 tsp. garlic, minced

- 1 ½ tsp. dried oregano
- 1/4 cup fresh lemon juice
- 1/4 cup olive oil
- 1/2 tsp. pepper
- 1 tsp. salt

Directions:

1. Add lamb chops in a mixing bowl. Add remaining ingredients over the lamb chops and coat well.
2. Arrange lamb chops on the air fryer oven tray and cook at 400°F for 5 minutes.
3. Turn lamb chops and cook for 5 more minutes.
4. Serve and enjoy.

Nutrition:

- Calories: 538
- Fat: 29.4 g
- Carbs: 1.3 g
- Protein: 64 g

82.   Herbed Lamb Chops

Preparation Time: 1 hour 10 minutes

Cooking Time: 13 minutes

Servings: 4

Ingredients:

- 1 lb. lamb chops, pastured

For the Marinate:

- 2 tbsp. lemon juice
- 1 tsp. dried rosemary
- 1 tsp. salt
- 1 tsp. dried thyme
- 1 tsp. coriander
- 1 tsp. dried oregano
- 2 tbsp. olive oil

Directions:

1. Prepare the marinade and for this, place all its ingredients in a bowl and whisk until combined.
2. Pour the marinade into a large plastic bag, add lamb chops in it, seal the bag, then turn it upside down to coat lamb chops with the marinade and let it in the refrigerator for a minimum of 1 hour.
3. Then switch on the air fryer, insert fryer basket, grease it with olive oil, then shut with its lid, set the fryer at 390°F, and preheat for 5 minutes.
4. Open the fryer, add marinated lamb chops in it, close with its lid and cook for 8 minutes until nicely golden and cooked, turning the lamb chops halfway through the frying.
5. When the air fryer beeps, open its lid, transfer lamb chops to a plate and serve.

Nutrition:

- Calories: 177.4

- Carbs: 1.7 g
- Fat: 8 g
- Protein: 23.4 g
- Fiber: 0.5 g

83.   Spicy Lamb Sirloin Steak

Preparation Time: 40 minutes

Cooking Time: 20 minutes

Servings: 4

Ingredients:

- 1 lb. lamb sirloin steaks, pastured, boneless

For the Marinade:

- 1/2 white onion, peeled
- 1 tsp. ground fennel
- 5 garlic cloves, peeled
- 4 slices ginger
- 1 tsp. salt
- 1/2 tsp. ground cardamom
- 1 tsp. garam masala
- 1 tsp. ground cinnamon
- 1 tsp. cayenne pepper

Directions:

1. Place all the ingredients for the marinade in a food processor and then pulse until well blended.

2. Make cuts in the lamb chops by using a knife, then place them in a large bowl and add prepared marinade in it.

3. Mix well until lamb chops are coated with the marinade and let them in the refrigerator for a minimum of 30 minutes.

4. Then switch on the air fryer, insert fryer basket, grease it with olive oil, then shut with its lid, set the fryer at 330°F, and preheat for 5 minutes.

5. Open the fryer, add lamb chops in it, close with its lid and cook for 15 minutes until nicely golden and cooked, flipping the steaks halfway through the frying.

6. When the air fryer beeps, open its lid, transfer lamb steaks to a plate and serve.

Nutrition:

- Calories: 182
- Carbs: 3 g
- Fat: 7 g
- Protein: 24 g
- Fiber: 1 g

84.   Garlic Rosemary Lamb Chops

Preparation Time: 1 hour 10 minutes

Cooking Time: 12 minutes

Servings: 4

Ingredients:

- 4 lamb chops, pastured
- 1 tsp. ground black pepper
- 2 tsp. minced garlic
- 1 ½ tsp. salt
- 2 tsp. olive oil
- 4 garlic cloves, peeled
- 4 rosemary sprigs

Directions:

1. Take the fryer pan, place lamb chops in it, season the top with ½ tsp. black pepper and ¾ tsp. salt, then drizzle evenly with oil and spread with 1 tsp. minced garlic.
2. Add garlic cloves and rosemary and then let the lamb chops marinate in the pan into the refrigerator for a minimum of 1 hour.
3. Then switch on the air fryer, insert fryer pan, then shut with its lid, set the fryer at 360°F, and cook for 6 minutes.
4. Flip the lamb chops, season them with remaining salt and black pepper, add remaining minced garlic, and continue cooking for 6 minutes or until lamb chops are cooked.
5. When the air fryer beeps, open its lid, transfer lamb chops to a plate and serve.

Nutrition:

- Calories: 616
- Carbs: 1 g
- Fat: 28 g
- Protein: 83 g

- Fiber: 0.3 g

85.   Cherry-Glazed Lamb Chops

Preparation Time: 10 minutes

Cooking Time: 20 minutes

Servings: 4

Ingredients:

- 4 (4 oz./113 g) lamb chops
- 1½ tsp. chopped fresh rosemary
- 1/4 tsp. salt
- 1/4 tsp. freshly ground black pepper
- 1 cup frozen cherries, thawed
- 1/4 cup dry red wine
- 2 tbsp. orange juice
- 1 tsp. extra-virgin olive oil

Directions:

1. Season the lamb chops with rosemary, salt, and pepper.
2. In a small saucepan over medium-low heat, combine the cherries, red wine, and orange juice, and simmer, stirring regularly, until the sauce thickens, 8 to 10 minutes.
3. Heat a large skillet over medium-high heat. When the pan is hot, add the olive oil to lightly coat the bottom.

4. Cook the lamb chops for 3 to 4 minutes on each side until well-browned yet medium-rare.

5. Serve topped with the cherry glaze.

Nutrition:

- Calories: 356
- Fat: 27 g
- Protein: 20 g
- Carbs: 6 g
- Sugars: 4 g
- Fiber: 1 g
- Sodium: 199 mg

86. Lamb and Vegetable Stew

Preparation Time: 10 minutes

Cooking Time: 3−6 hours

Servings: 3

Ingredients:

- 1 lb. (454 g) boneless lamb stew meat
- 1 lb. (454 g) turnips, peeled, and chopped
- 1 fennel bulb, trimmed and thinly sliced
- 10 oz. (283 g) mushrooms, sliced
- 1 onion, diced
- 3 garlic cloves, minced
- 2 cups low-sodium chicken broth
- 2 tbsp. tomato paste
- 1/4 cup dry red wine (optional)
- 1 tsp. chopped fresh thyme
- 1/2 tsp. salt
- 1/4 tsp. freshly ground black pepper
- Chopped fresh parsley to garnish

Directions:

1. In a slow cooker, combine the lamb, turnips, fennel, mushrooms, onion, garlic, chicken broth, tomato paste, red wine (if using), thyme, salt, and pepper.

2. Cover and cook on high for 3 hours or on low for 6 hours. When the meat is tender and falling apart, garnish with parsley and serve.

3. If you don't have a slow cooker, in a large pot, heat 2 teaspoons of olive oil over medium heat, and sear the lamb on all sides. Remove from the pot and set aside.

4. Add the turnips, fennel, mushrooms, onion, and garlic to the pot, and cook for 3 to 4 minutes until the vegetables begin to soften.

5. Add the chicken broth, tomato paste, red wine (if using), thyme, salt, pepper, and browned lamb. Bring to a boil, then reduce the heat to low. Simmer for 1½ to 2 hours until the meat is tender. Garnish with parsley and serve.

Nutrition:

- Calories: 303
- Fat: 7 g
- Protein: 32 g

- Carbs: 27 g
- Sugars: 7 g
- Fiber: 4 g
- Sodium: 310 mg

87.   Lime-Parsley Lamb Cutlets

Preparation Time: 10 minutes

Cooking Time: 10 minutes

Servings: 4

Ingredients:

- 1/4 cup extra-virgin olive oil
- 1/4 cup freshly squeezed lime juice
- 2 tbsp. lime zest
- 2 tbsp. chopped fresh parsley
- Pinch sea salt
- Pinch freshly ground black pepper
- 12 lamb cutlets (about 1½ lb./680 g total)

Directions:

1. In a medium bowl, whisk together the oil, lime juice, zest, parsley, salt, and pepper.
2. Transfer the marinade to a resealable plastic bag.
3. Add the cutlets to the bag and remove as much air as possible before sealing.
4. Marinate the lamb in the refrigerator for about 4 hours, turning the bag several times.
5. Preheat the oven to broil.
6. Remove the chops from the bag and arrange them on an aluminum foil-lined baking sheet. Discard the marinade.
7. Broil the chops for 4 minutes per side for medium doneness.
8. Let the chops rest for 5 minutes before serving.

Nutrition:

- Calories: 413
- Fat: 29 g
- Protein: 31 g
- Carbs: 1 g
- Sugars: 0 g
- Fiber: 0 g
- Sodium: 100 mg

CHAPTER 12. DINNER RECIPES

62.   Oven-Baked Potatoes and Green Beans

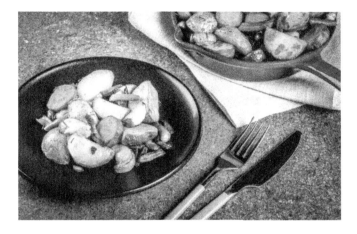

Preparation time: 10 minutes

Cooking time: 30 minutes

Servings: 4

Ingredients:

- 1/2 lb. green beans
- 1/2 lb. potatoes, peeled and sliced into chunks
- 2 tsp. extra-virgin olive oil
- 1/2 tsp. garlic powder
- 2 tsp. Dijon mustard
- Sea salt along with fresh ground black pepper as needed

Directions:

1. Preheat oven to 375°F.
2. Mix your chunks of potatoes with oil and mustard. Spread prepared potato chunks over a baking sheet. Bake for 15 minutes to make the first layer.
3. Add your green beans, garlic powder, sea salt, and black pepper to your potatoes and toss—Bake for an additional 15 minutes. Serve and enjoy!

Nutrition:

- Calories: 35
- Carbohydrates: 5.5 g
- Protein: 1.3 g
- Fat: 0.3 g

63.   Hummus and Salad Pita Flats

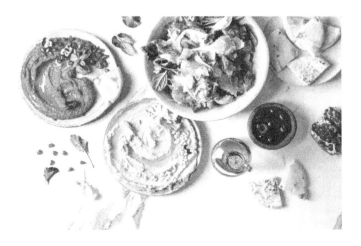

Preparation time: 15 minutes

Cooking time: 0 minute

Servings: 2

Ingredients:

- 2 oz. whole-wheat pitas
- 8 black olives, pitted
- 1/4 cup sweet roasted red pepper hummus
- 2 large eggs
- 2 tsp. spring mix
- 1 tsp. dried oregano
- 2 tsp. extra-virgin olive oil

Directions:

1. Heat your pitas according to the package instructions.
2. Spread the hummus over the pitas.
3. Top pitas with hard-boiled eggs, dried oregano, and olives.
4. Add the spring mix and extra-virgin olive oil. Serve and enjoy!

Nutrition:

- Calories: 250
- Carbohydrates: 50 g
- Protein: 8 g
- Fat: 2 g

64.   Lettuce Salad with Lemon

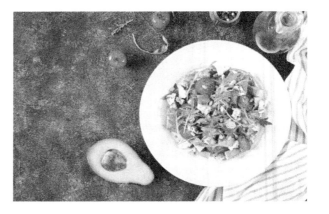

Preparation time: 5 minutes

Cooking time: 5 minutes

Servings: 2

Ingredients:

- 2 oz. arugula
- 1/2 head Romaine lettuce, chopped
- 1 avocado, pitted and sliced
- 2 tsp. extra-virgin olive oil
- 1 tbsp. lemon juice
- Sea salt along with fresh ground black pepper as needed

Directions:

1. Whisk your torn arugula, lemon juice, chopped avocado, olive oil, sea salt, and pepper.
2. Add the chopped lettuce and toss to coat. Serve and enjoy!

Nutrition:

- Calories: 15
- Carbohydrates: 1 g
- Protein: 2 g
- Fat: 2 g

65. Pork Chops and Butternut Squash Salad

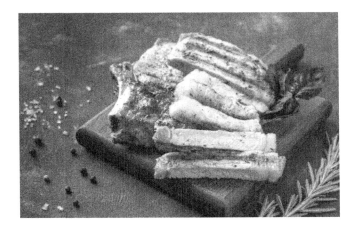

Preparation time: 20 minutes

Cooking time: 25 minutes

Servings: 4

Ingredients:

- 4 boneless pork chops
- 1 1/2 tbsp. fresh lemon juice
- 1 package pomegranate seeds
- 1 package baby arugula
- 3 cups butternut squash, peeled and cubed
- 1/2 cup pine nuts
- 2 tbsp. extra-virgin olive oil (divided)
- 2 garlic cloves, minced
- 6 tbsp. balsamic vinaigrette
- Sea salt along with fresh ground black pepper as needed

Directions:

1. Preheat your oven to 475°F.
2. Combine a tbsp. olive oil, minced garlic, and lemon juice.
3. Mix your pork chops with an oil mixture, sprinkle the top of the chops with sea salt and pepper.
4. Mix squash and 1 tbsp. oil, sprinkle with salt and pepper.
5. Place your pork chops onto a baking sheet, add place cubed squash around the chops. Bake for 25 minutes, then turn chops.
6. Toast your pine nuts for about 5 minutes in a small pan over medium-high heat.
7. Combine your squash, pine nuts, arugula, and pomegranate seeds. Drizzle with balsamic vinaigrette and toss. Serve and enjoy!

Nutrition:

- Calories: 310
- Carbohydrates: 2 g
- Protein: 20 g
- Fat: 17 g

66.   Low Carb Stuffed Peppers

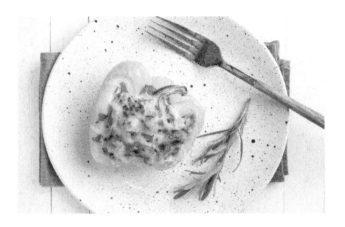

Preparation time: 15 minutes

Cooking time: 30 minutes

Servings: 4

Ingredients:

- 1 onion, diced
- 2 lb. Ground steak
- 4 green bell peppers, seeds removed and cut in half
- Sea salt along with black ground pepper
- 1 tbsp. Worcestershire sauce
- 2 tsp. garlic, minced
- 4 slices of mozzarella cheese
- 2 tbsp. oil

Directions:

1. Heat your oil, add diced onions and minced garlic along with some salt and pepper in the pan over medium-high heat.
2. Add diced steak pieces into the pan along with Worcestershire sauce and cook for 5 minutes.
3. Add cooked steak and other ingredients into a bowl and combine (except cheese slices and pepper halves).
4. Fill the pepper halves with a steak mixture and top with a thin piece of mozzarella cheese on top of each half pepper.
5. Place the peppers into a baking pan and bake for 3o minutes. Serve and enjoy!

Nutrition:

- Calories: 320
- Carbohydrates: 10 g
- Protein: 40 g
- Fat: 19 g

67.   Chicken Cordon Bleu

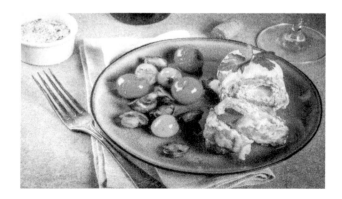

Preparation time: 20 minutes

Cooking time: 25 minutes

Servings: 4

Ingredients:

- 8 chicken breasts, boneless and skinless
- 1/2 cup fat-free sour cream
- 2/3 cup skim milk
- 1 1/2 cups mozzarella cheese, grated
- 8 slices of ham
- 1 cup corn flakes, crushed
- 1 can low-fat condensed cream of chicken soup
- 1 tsp. lemon juice
- 1 tsp. paprika
- 1/2 tsp. garlic powder
- 1/2 tsp. black pepper
- 1/4 tsp. sea salt
- Non-stick cooking spray as needed

Directions:

1. Heat your oven to 350°F. Spray a 13×9 baking dish lightly with cooking spray.
2. Flatten the chicken breasts to 1/4-inch thick. Sprinkle with pepper and top with a slice of ham and 3 tbsp. cheese down the middle. Roll up, and tuck ends under and secure with toothpicks.
3. Pour the milk into a shallow bowl. In another bowl, combine corn flakes and seasoning. Dip the chicken into milk, roll in the cornflake mixture, and then place on a prepared baking dish.
4. Bake for 30 minutes or until your chicken is cooked through.
5. In a small pan, whisk the soup, lemon juice, and sour cream until well combined. Cook over medium heat until hot.
6. Remove the toothpicks from your chicken and place them onto serving plates. Top with sauce, serve and enjoy!

Nutrition:

- Calories: 382
- Carbohydrates: 9 g
- Protein: 50 g
- Fats: 14 g

68.   Beef Goulash

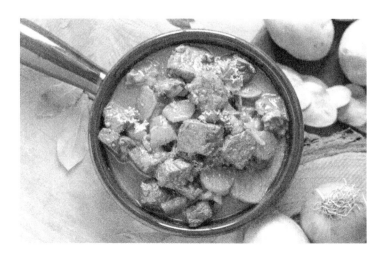

Preparation time: 15 minutes

Cooking time: 1 hour

Servings: 4

Ingredients:

- 2 lb. chuck steak, trim the fat and cut into bite-sized pieces
- 1 orange pepper, chopped
- 1 red pepper, chopped
- 1 green pepper, chopped
- 3 onions, quartered
- 3 garlic cloves, diced fine
- 1 cup low-sodium beef broth
- 1 can tomatoes, chopped
- 2 tbsp. tomato paste
- 3 cups water
- 2 bay leaves
- 1 tbsp. paprika
- 1 tbsp. olive oil
- 2 tsp. hot smoked paprika
- Sea salt and black pepper to taste

Directions:

1. Heat your oil in a soup pot over medium-high heat. Add the steak and cook until browned, stirring often.
2. Add your onions, and continue to cook for another 5 minutes or until soft. Add the garlic and cook for another minute, stirring often.

3. Add your remaining ingredients, then bring to a boil. Reduce the heat to a low simmer for 50 minutes, stirring occasionally. The Goulash is done when the steak is tender. Stir well, then add to serving bowls and enjoy!

Nutrition:

- Calories: 413
- Carbohydrates: 14 g
- Protein: 53 g
- Fats: 15 g

69.   Cajun Beef and Rice Skillet

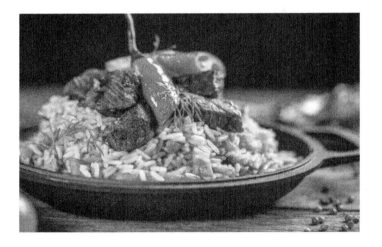

Preparation time: 10 minutes

Cooking time: 25 minutes

Servings: 4

Ingredients:

- 2 cups cauliflower rice, cooked
- 3/4 lb. lean ground beef
- 1 red bell pepper, sliced thin
- 1 jalapeno pepper, with seeds removed and diced fine
- 1 celery stalk, sliced thin
- 1/2 yellow onion, diced
- 1/4 cup parsley, fresh diced
- 4 tsp. Cajun seasoning
- 1/2 cup low-sodium beef broth

Directions:

1. Place the beef along with 1 1/2 tsp. Cajun seasoning into a large skillet over medium-high heat.
2. Add the vegetables, except cauliflower and remaining Cajun seasoning. Cook, occasionally stirring, for about 8 minutes or until vegetables are tender.
3. Add the broth and stir, and cook for 3 minutes or until the mixture has thickened. Stir in your cauliflower rice and cook until heated through. Remove from heat and add to serving bowls, then top with parsley, serve and enjoy!

Nutrition:

- Calories: 198
- Carbohydrates: 8 g
- Protein: 28 g
- Fats: 6 g

70.   Cheesy Beef and Noodles

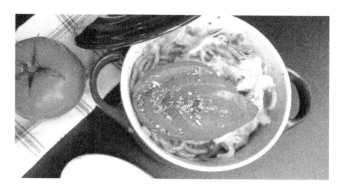

Preparation time: 10 minutes

Cooking time: 15 minutes

Servings: 4

Ingredients:

- 1 lb. lean ground beef
- 2 cups mozzarella cheese, grated
- 1 onion, diced
- 1/2 cup + 2 tbsp. fresh parsley, diced
- 1 package Fettuccine noodles
- 2 tbsp. tomato paste
- 1 tbsp. Worcestershire sauce
- 1 tbsp. extra-virgin olive oil
- 3 garlic cloves, minced
- 1 tsp. red pepper flakes
- Sea salt and black pepper to taste
- 1/2 cup water

Directions:

1. Heat your oil in a large skillet placed over medium-high heat. Add the beef and cook while breaking up with the spatula for about 2 minutes.
2. Cook the noodles according to package instructions.
3. Lower the heat of your skillet to medium, then season with salt and pepper. Stir in your garlic, pepper flakes, onion, tomato paste, 1/2 cup parsley, Worcestershire sauce, and 1/2 cup of water. Bring to a simmer while occasionally stirring for about 8 minutes.
4. Stir in the cooked noodles and continue to cook for another 2 minutes. Stir in 1 cup of cheese over the top and cover with a lid until cheese melts. Serve garnishing with remaining parsley, and enjoy!

Nutrition:

- Calories: 372
- Carbohydrates: 7 g
- Protein: 44 g
- Fats: 18g

71. Bone Broth

Preparation time: 10 minutes

Cooking time: 60 minutes

Servings: 2

Ingredients:

- 1 chicken carcass and dripping or 1 large marrow bone
- 1 chopped onion
- 1 stalk chopped celery
- 1tbsp. minced garlic
- 1tbsp. bouillon powder
- 2 cups water

Directions:

1. Place the chicken, onion, and celery in your Instant Pot.
2. Cover with 2 cups of water.
3. Seal and cook on Manual, high pressure, for 60 minutes.
4. Release the pressure naturally.
5. Strain the solids out.
6. Add the garlic and bouillon.

Nutrition:

- Calories: 38
- Carbohydrates: 2 g
- Protein: 3 g
- Fat: 2 g
- Sugar: 0 g

72. Tofu Mushrooms

Preparation time: 5 minutes

Cooking time: 10minutes

Servings: 3

Ingredients:

- 1 block tofu
- 1 cup mushrooms
- 4 tbsp. butter
- 4 tbsp. parmesan cheese
- Salt to taste
- Ground black pepper to taste

Directions:

1. Toss tofu cubes with melted butter, salt, and black pepper in a mixing bowl.
2. Sauté the tofu within 5 minutes. Stir in cheese and mushrooms.
3. Sauté for another 5 minutes.

Nutrition:

- Calories: 211
- Carbohydrates: 2 g
- Protein: 11.5 g
- Fat: 18.5 g
- Cholesterol: 51 mg
- Sodium: 346 mg

73.   Onion Tofu

Preparation time: 8 minutes

Cooking time: 5 minutes

Servings: 3

Ingredients:

- 2 blocks of tofu
- 2 onions
- 2 tbsp. butter
- 1 cup cheddar cheese
- Salt to taste
- Ground black pepper to taste

Directions:

1. Rub the tofu with salt and pepper in a bowl.
2. Add melted butter and onions to a skillet to sauté within 3 minutes.
3. Toss in tofu and stir cook for 2 minutes. Stir in cheese and cover the skillet for 5 minutes on low heat. Serve.

Nutrition:

- Calories: 184
- Carbohydrates: 6.3 g
- Protein: 12.2 g
- Fat: 12.7 g
- Sugar: 2.7 g
- Fiber: 1.6 g

74.   Spinach Rich Ballet

Preparation time: 5 minutes

Cooking time: 30minutes

Servings: 4

Ingredients:

- 1 1/2 lbs. baby spinach
- 8 tsp. coconut cream
- 14 oz. cauliflower
- 2 tbsp. unsalted butter
- Salt to taste
- Ground black pepper to taste

Directions:

1. Warm-up oven at 360°F.
2. Melt butter, then toss in spinach to sauté for 3 minutes.
3. Divide the spinach into four ramekins.
4. Divide cream, cauliflower, salt, and black pepper in the ramekins.
5. Bake within 25 minutes.

Nutrition:

- Calories: 188
- Carbohydrates: 4.9 g
- Protein: 14.6 g
- Fat: 12.5 g
- Cholesterol: 53 mg
- Sodium: 1098 mg

75.   Pepperoni Egg Omelet

Preparation time: 5 minutes

Cooking time: 20minutes

Servings: 4

Ingredients:

- 15 pepperonis
- 6 eggs
- 2 tbsp. butter
- 4 tbsp. coconut cream
- Salt and ground black pepper to taste

Directions:

1. Whisk eggs with pepperoni, cream, salt, and black pepper in a bowl.
2. Add 1/4 of the butter to a warm-up pan.
3. Now pour 1/4 of the batter in this melted butter and cook for 2 minutes on each side.

Nutrition:

- Calories: 141
- Protein: 8.9 g
- Fat: 11.3 g
- Cholesterol: 181 mg
- Sodium: 334 mg

76.   Nut Porridge

Preparation time: 10 minutes

Cooking time: 15 minutes

Servings: 4

Ingredients:

- 1 cup cashew nuts
- 1 cup pecan
- 2 tbsp. Stevia
- 4 tsp. coconut oil
- 2 cups water

Directions:

1. Grind the cashews and pecan in a processor.
2. Stir in Stevia, oil, and water. Add the mixture to a saucepan and cook within 5 minutes on high. Adjust on low within 10 minutes. Serve.

Nutrition:

- Calories: 260
- Carbohydrates: 12.7 g
- Protein: 5.6 g
- Fat: 22.9 g
- Sugar: 1.8 g
- Fiber: 1.4 g
- Sodium: 9 mg

77.   Parsley Soufflé

Preparation time: 5 minutes

Cooking time: 6 minutes

Servings: 1

Ingredients:

- 2 eggs
- 1 red chili pepper
- 2 tbsp. coconut cream
- 1 tbsp. parsley
- Salt to taste

Directions:

1. Blend all the Soufflé ingredients in a food processor.
2. Put it in the Soufflé dishes, then bake within 6 minutes at 390°F.

Nutrition:

- Calories: 108
- Carbohydrates: 1.1 g
- Protein: 6 g
- Fat: 9 g
- Cholesterol: 180 mg
- Sodium: 146 mg

78.   Eggs and Ham

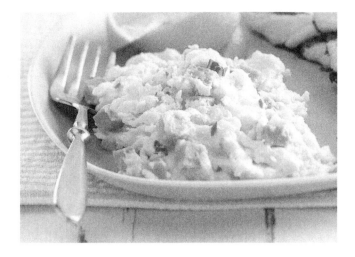

Preparation time: 25 minutes

Cooking time: 15 minutes

Servings: 4

Ingredients:

- 4 eggs
- 10 ham slices
- 4 tbsp. scallions
- A pinch of black pepper
- A pinch of sweet paprika
- 1 tbsp. melted ghee

Directions:

1. Grease a muffin pan with melted ghee.
2. Divide ham slices into each muffin mold to form your cups. In a bowl, mix eggs with scallions, pepper, and paprika and whisk well.

3. Divide this mix on top of the ham, introduce your ham cups in the oven at 400°F and bake for 15 minutes. Leave cups to cool down before dividing on plates and serving.

Nutrition:

- Calories: 250
- Carbohydrates: 6 g
- Protein: 12 g
- Fat: 10 g
- Fiber: 3 g

79.   Spicy Keto Chicken Wings

Preparation time: 20 minutes

Cooking time: 30 minutes

Servings: 4

Ingredients:

- 2 lbs. chicken wings
- 1 tsp. Cajun spice
- 2 tsp. smoked paprika
- 1/2 tsp. turmeric
- A dash of salt
- 2 tsp. baking powder
- A dash of pepper

Directions:

1. When you are all set, take out a mixing bowl and place all of the seasonings along with the baking powder. If you feel like it, you can adjust the seasoning levels however you would like.

2. Once these are set, go ahead, and throw the chicken wings in and coat evenly. If you have one, you'll want to place the wings on a wire rack that is placed over your baking tray. If not, you can just lay them across the baking sheet.

3. Now that your chicken wings are set, you are going to pop them into the stove for 30 minutes. By the end of this time, the tops of the wings should be crispy.

4. If they are, take them out from the oven and flip them so that you can bake the other side. You will want to cook these for an additional 30 minutes.

5. Finally, take the tray from the oven and allow it to cool slightly before serving up your spiced keto wings. For additional flavor, serve with any of your favorite, keto-friendly dipping sauce.

Nutrition:

- Calories: 380
- Carbohydrates: 1 g
- Proteins: 60 g
- Fats: 7 g

80. Sesame-Crusted Tuna with Green Beans

Preparation time: 15 minutes

Cooking time: 5 minutes

Servings: 4

Ingredients:

- 1/4 cup white sesame seeds
- 1/4 cup black sesame seeds
- 4 (6 oz.) ahi tuna steaks
- Salt and pepper to taste
- 1 tbsp. olive oil
- 1 tbsp. coconut oil
- 2 cups green beans

Directions:

1. In a shallow dish, mix the 2 kinds of sesame seeds.

2. Season the tuna with pepper and salt.

3. Dredge the tuna in a mixture of sesame seeds.

4. Heat up to high heat the olive oil in a skillet, then add the tuna.

5. Cook for 1 to 2 minutes until it turns seared, then sear on the other side.

6. Remove the tuna from the skillet and let the tuna rest while using the coconut oil to heat the skillet.

7. Fry the green beans in the oil for 5 minutes then use sliced tuna to eat.

Nutrition:

- Calories: 380
- Carbohydrates: 8 g
- Protein: 44.5 g
- Fat: 19 g
- Fiber: 3 g

81. Grilled Salmon and Zucchini with Mango Sauce

Preparation time: 5 minutes

Cooking time: 10 minutes

Servings: 4

Ingredients:

- 4 (6 oz.) boneless salmon fillets
- 1 tbsp. olive oil
- Salt and pepper to taste
- 1 large zucchini, sliced in coins
- 2 tbsp. fresh lemon juice
- 1/2 cup chopped mango
- 1/4 cup fresh chopped cilantro
- 1 tsp. lemon zest
- 1/2 cup canned coconut milk
- Cooking spray

Directions:

1. Preheat a grill pan to heat, and sprinkle with cooking spray liberally.
2. Brush with olive oil to the salmon and season with salt and pepper.
3. Apply lemon juice to the zucchini, and season with salt and pepper.
4. Put the zucchini and salmon fillets on the grill pan.
5. Cook for 5 minutes then turn all over and cook for another 5 minutes.
6. Combine the remaining ingredients in a blender and combine to create a sauce.
7. Serve the side-drizzled salmon filets with mango sauce and zucchini.

Nutrition:

- Calories: 350
- Carbohydrates: 8 g
- Protein: 35 g
- Fat: 21.5 g
- Sugar

CHAPTER 13. BEEF RECIPES FOR DINNER

108.   Meatloaf Slider Wraps

Preparation Time: 15 minutes

Cooking Time: 10 minutes

Servings: 2

Ingredients:

- 1 pound ground beef, grass-fed
- 1/2 cup almond flour
- 1/4 cup coconut flour
- 1/2 tbsp. minced garlic
- 1/4 cup chopped white onion
- 1 tsp. Italian seasoning
- 1/2 tsp. sea salt
- 1/2 tsp. dried tarragon
- 1/2 tsp. ground black pepper
- 1 tbsp. Worcestershire sauce
- 1/4 cup ketchup
- 2 eggs, pastured, beaten
- 1 head of lettuce

Directions:

1. Place all the ingredients in a bowl, stir well, then shape the mixture into 2-inch diameters and 1-inch thick patties and refrigerate them for 10 minutes.

2. Meanwhile, switch on the air fryer, insert the fryer basket, grease it with olive oil, then shut with its lid, set the fryer at 360°F, and preheat for 10 minutes.

3. Open the fryer, add patties to it in a single layer, close with its lid and cook for 10 minutes until nicely golden and cooked, flipping the patties halfway through the frying.

4. When the air fryer beeps, open its lid and transfer patties to a plate.

5. Wrap each patty in lettuce and serve.

Nutrition:

- Calories: 228
- Carbs: 6 g
- Fat: 16 g
- Protein: 13 g
- Fiber: 2 g

109.   Double Cheeseburger

Preparation Time: 5 minutes

Cooking Time: 18 minutes

Servings: 1

Ingredients:

- 2 beef patties, pastured
- 1/8 tsp. onion powder
- 2 slices of mozzarella cheese, low-fat
- 1/8 tsp. ground black pepper

- 1/8 tsp. salt
- 2 tbsp of olive oil

Directions:

1. Switch on the air fryer, insert the basket, grease it with olive oil, then shut with its lid, set the fryer at 370ºF and preheat for 5 minutes.
2. Meanwhile, season the patties well with onion powder, black pepper, and salt.
3. Open the fryer, add beef patties in it, close with its lid and cook for 12 minutes until nicely golden and cooked, flipping the patties halfway through the frying.
4. Then top the patties with a cheese slice and continue cooking for 1 minute or until cheese melts.
5. Serve straight away.

Nutrition:

- Calories: 670
- Carbs: 0 g
- Fat: 50 g
- Protein: 39 g
- Fiber: 0 g

110.   Beef Schnitzel

Preparation Time: 10 minutes

Cooking Time: 15 minutes

Servings: 1

Ingredients:

- 1 lean beef schnitzel
- 2 tbsp. olive oil
- 1/4 cup breadcrumbs
- 1 egg
- 1 lemon and salad greens to serve

Directions:

1. Let the air fryer heat to 180ºC.
2. In a big bowl, add breadcrumbs and oil, mix well until it forms a crumbly mixture.
3. Dip beef steak in whisked egg and coat in breadcrumbs mixture.
4. Place the breaded beef in the air fryer and cook at 180C for 15 minutes or more until fully cooked through.
5. Take out from the air fryer and serve with the side of salad greens and lemon.

Nutrition:

- Calories: 340
- Proteins: 20 g
- Carbs: 14 g
- Fat: 10 g
- Fiber: 7 g

111.   Steak with Asparagus Bundles

Preparation Time: 20 minutes

Cooking Time: 30 minutes

Servings: 2

Ingredients:

- Olive oil spray
- 2 lb. flank steak, cut into 6 pieces
- Kosher salt and black pepper
- 2 cloves minced garlic
- 4 cups asparagus
- 1/2 Tamari sauce
- 3 bell peppers sliced thinly
- 1/3 cup beef broth
- 1 tbsp. unsalted butter
- 1/4 cup balsamic vinegar

Directions:

1. Sprinkle salt and pepper on steak and rub.
2. In a Ziploc bag, add garlic and Tamari sauce, then add steak, toss well and seal the bag.
3. Let it marinate for 1 hour or overnight.
4. Equally, place bell peppers and asparagus in the center of the steak.
5. Roll the steak around the vegetables and secure well with toothpicks.
6. Preheat the air fryer.
7. Drizzle the steak with olive oil spray. And place steaks in the air fryer.
8. Cook for 15 minutes at 400°F or more until steaks are cooked.
9. Take the steak out from the air fryer and let it rest for 5 minutes.
10. Remove steak bundles and allow them to rest for 5 minutes before serving and slicing.
11. In the meantime, add butter, balsamic vinegar, and broth over medium flame. Mix well and reduce it by half. Add salt and pepper to taste.
12. Pour over steaks right before serving.

Nutrition:

- Calories: 471
- Proteins: 29 g
- Carbs: 20 g
- Fat: 15 g

112.   Hamburgers

Preparation Time: 5 minutes

Cooking Time: 6 minutes

Servings: 4

Ingredients:

- 4 buns
- 4 cups lean ground beef chuck
- Salt to taste
- 4 slices any cheese
- Black Pepper to taste
- 2 sliced tomatoes
- 1 head of lettuce
- Ketchup for dressing

Directions:

1. Let the air fryer preheat to 350°F.

2. In a bowl, add lean ground beef, pepper, and salt. Mix well and form patties.

3. Put them in the air fryer in one layer only, cook for 6 minutes, flip them halfway through. 1 minute before you take out the patties, add cheese on top.

4. When cheese is melted, take it out from the air fryer.

5. Add ketchup or any dressing to your buns; add tomatoes, lettuce, and patties.

6. Serve hot.

Nutrition:

- Calories: 520
- Carbs: 22 g
- Protein: 31 g
- Fat: 34 g

113. Beef Steak Kabobs with Vegetables

Preparation Time: 30 minutes

Cooking Time: 10 minutes

Servings: 4

Ingredients:

- 2 tbsp. light soy sauce
- 4 cups lean beef chuck ribs, cut into 1-inch pieces
- 1/3 cup low-fat sour cream
- 1/2 onion

- 8 6-inch skewers
- 1 bell pepper
- Black pepper
- Yogurt for dipping

Directions:

1. In a mixing bowl, add soy sauce and sour cream, mix well. Add the lean beef chunks, coat well, and let it marinate for half an hour or more.

2. Cut onion, bell pepper into 1-inch pieces. In water, soak skewers for 10 minutes.

3. Add onions, bell peppers, and beef on skewers; alternatively, sprinkle with black pepper.

4. Let it cook for 10 minutes in a preheated air fryer at 400°F, flip halfway through.

5. Serve with yogurt dipping sauce.

Nutrition:

- Calories: 268
- Proteins: 20 g
- Carbs: 15 g
- Fat: 10 g

114. Rib-Eye Steak

Preparation Time: 5 minutes

Cooking Time: 14 minutes

Servings: 2

Ingredients:

- 2 lean ribeye steaks medium-sized
- Salt and freshly ground black pepper to taste
- Microgreen salad to serve

Directions:

1. Let the air fryer preheat at 400°F. Pat dry steaks with paper towels.
2. Use any spice blend or just salt and pepper on steaks.
3. Generously on both sides of the steak.
4. Put steaks in the air fryer basket. Cook according to the rareness you want. Or cook for 14 minutes and flip after halftime.
5. Take out from the air fryer and let it rest for about 5 minutes.
6. Serve with microgreen salad.

Nutrition:

- Calories: 470
- Protein: 45 g
- Fat: 31 g
- Carbs: 23 g

115.   Bunless Sloppy Joes

Preparation Time: 15 minutes

Cooking Time: 40 minutes

Servings: 2

Ingredients:

- 6 small sweet potatoes
- 1 pound (454 g) lean ground beef
- 1 onion, finely chopped
- 1 carrot, finely chopped
- 1/4 cup finely chopped mushrooms
- 1/4 cup finely chopped red bell pepper
- 3 garlic cloves, minced
- 2 tsp. Worcestershire sauce
- 1 tbsp. white wine vinegar
- 1 (15 oz./425 g) can low-sodium tomato sauce
- 2 tbsp. tomato paste

Directions:

1. Preheat the air fryer oven to 400°F (205°C).
2. Place the sweet potatoes in a single layer in a baking dish. Bake for 25 to 40 minutes, depending on the size, until they are soft and cooked through.
3. While the sweet potatoes are baking in a large skillet, cook the beef over medium heat until it's browned, breaking it apart into small pieces as you stir.
4. Add the onion, carrot, mushrooms, bell pepper, and garlic, and saute briefly for 1 minute.
5. Stir in the Worcestershire sauce, vinegar, tomato sauce, and tomato paste. Bring to a simmer, reduce the heat, and cook for 5 minutes for the flavors to meld.
6. Scoop ½ cup of the meat mixture on top of each baked potato and serve.

Nutrition:

- Calories: 372
- Fat: 19 g
- Protein: 16 g
- Carbs: 34 g
- Sugars: 13 g
- Fiber: 6 g
- Sodium: 161 mg

116.   Beef Curry

Preparation Time: 15 minutes

Cooking Time: 10 minutes

Servings: 2

Ingredients:

- 1 tbsp. extra-virgin olive oil
- 1 small onion, thinly sliced
- 2 tsp. minced fresh ginger
- 3 garlic cloves, minced
- 2 tsp. ground coriander
- 1 tsp. ground cumin
- 1 jalapeño or serrano pepper, split lengthwise but not all the way through
- 1/4 tsp. ground turmeric
- 1/4 tsp. salt
- 1 lb. (454 g) grass-fed sirloin tip steak, top round steak, or top sirloin steak, cut into bite-size pieces
- 2 tbsp. chopped fresh cilantro

- 1/4 cup water

Directions:

1. In an air fryer oven, heat the oil over medium-high.
2. Add the onion, and cook for 3 to 5 minutes until browned and softened. Add the ginger and garlic, stirring continuously until fragrant, about 30 seconds.
3. In a small bowl, mix the coriander, cumin, jalapeño, turmeric, and salt. Add the spice mixture to the skillet and stir continuously for 1 minute. Deglaze the skillet with about ¼ cup of water.
4. Add the beef and stir continuously for about 5 minutes until well-browned yet still medium-rare. Remove the jalapeño. Serve topped with cilantro.

Nutrition:

- Calories: 140
- Fat: 7 g
- Protein: 18 g
- Carbs: 3 g
- Sugars: 1 g
- Fiber: 1 g
- Sodium: 141 mg

117.   Asian Grilled Beef Salad

Preparation Time: 15 minutes

Cooking Time: 15 minutes

Servings: 4

Ingredients:

Dressing:

- 1/4 cup freshly squeezed lime juice
- 1 tbsp. low-sodium tamari or gluten-free soy sauce
- 1 tbsp. extra-virgin olive oil
- 1 garlic clove, minced
- 1 tsp. honey
- 1/4 tsp. red pepper flakes

Salad:

- 1 lb. (454 g) grass-fed flank steak
- 1/4 tsp. salt
- Pinch freshly ground black pepper
- 6 cups chopped leaf lettuce
- 1 cucumber, halved lengthwise and thinly cut into half-moons
- 1/2 small red onion, sliced
- 1 carrot, cut into ribbons
- 1/4 cup chopped fresh cilantro

Directions:

Make the Dressing:

1. In a small bowl, whisk together the lime juice, tamari, olive oil, garlic, honey, and red pepper flakes. Set aside.

Make the Salad:

1. Season the beef on both sides with salt and pepper.
2. Preheat the air fryer oven to 400°F (205°C).
3. Cook the beef for 3 to 6 minutes per side, depending on preferred doneness. Set aside, tented with aluminum foil, for 10 minutes.
4. In a large bowl, toss the lettuce, cucumber, onion, carrot, and cilantro.
5. Slice the beef thinly against the grain and transfer to the salad bowl.
6. Drizzle with the dressing and toss. Serve.

Nutrition:

- Calories: 231
- Fat: 10 g
- Protein: 26 g
- Carbs: 10 g
- Sugars: 4 g
- Fiber: 2 g
- Sodium: 349 mg

118. Sunday Pot Roast

Preparation Time: 10 minutes

Cooking Time: 1 hour 45 minutes

Servings: 4

Ingredients:

- 1 (3 to 4 lb./1.4 to 1.8 kg) beef rump roast
- 2 tsp. kosher salt, divided
- 2 tbsp. avocado oil

- 1 large onion, coarsely chopped (about 1½ cup)
- 4 large carrots, each cut into 4 pieces
- 1 tbsp. minced garlic
- 3 cups low-sodium beef broth
- 1 tsp. freshly ground black pepper
- 1 tbsp. dried parsley
- 2 tbsp. all-purpose flour

Directions:

1. Rub the roast all over with 1 tsp. salt.
2. Preheat the air fryer oven to 400°F (205°C).
3. Pour in the avocado oil. Carefully, place the roast in the pot and sear it for 6 to 9 minutes on each side. (You want a dark caramelized crust.) Hit "Cancel."
4. Transfer the roast from the pot to a plate.
5. In order, put the onion, carrots, and garlic in the pot. Place the roast on top of the vegetables along with any juices that accumulated on the plate.
6. In a medium bowl, whisk together the broth, remaining 1 tsp. of salt, pepper, and parsley. Pour the broth mixture over the roast.
7. Close and lock the lid of the air fryer. Set the valve to sealing.
8. Cook on high pressure for 1 hour and 30 minutes.
9. When the cooking is completed, hit "Cancel" and allow the pressure to release naturally.
10. Once the pin drops, unlock and remove the lid.
11. Using large slotted spoons, transfer the roast and vegetables to a serving platter while you make the gravy.
12. Using a large spoon or fat separator, remove the fat from the juices in the pot. Set the electric pressure cooker to the "Sauté" setting and bring the liquid to a boil.
13. In a small bowl, whisk together the flour and 4 tablespoons of water to make a slurry. Pour the slurry into the pot, whisking occasionally, until the gravy is the thickness you like. Season with salt and pepper, if necessary.
14. Serve the meat and carrots with the gravy.

Nutrition:

- Calories: 245
- Fat: 10 g
- Protein: 33 g
- Carbs: 6 g
- Sugars: 2 g
- Fiber: 1 g
- Sodium: 397 mg

119. Beef Burrito Bowl

Preparation Time: 5 minutes

Cooking Time: 10 minutes

Servings: 4

Ingredients:

- 1 lb. (454 g) 93% lean ground beef
- 1 cup canned low-sodium black beans, drained, and rinsed

- 1/4 tsp. ground cumin
- 1/4 tsp. chili powder
- 1/4 tsp. garlic powder
- 1/4 tsp. onion powder
- 1/4 tsp. salt
- 1 head romaine or preferred lettuce, shredded
- 2 medium tomatoes, chopped
- 1 cup shredded Cheddar cheese or packaged cheese blend

Directions:

1. Preheat the air fryer oven to 400°F (205°C).
2. Put the beef, beans, cumin, chili powder, garlic powder, onion powder, and salt into the skillet, and cook for 8 to 10 minutes until cooked through. Stir occasionally.
3. Divide the lettuce evenly between four bowls. Add 1/4 of the beef mixture to each bowl and top with 1/4 of the tomatoes and cheese.

Nutrition:

- Calories: 351
- Fat: 18 g
- Protein: 35 g
- Carbs: 14 g
- Sugars: 4 g
- Fiber: 6 g
- Sodium: 424 mg

120.   Beef and Pepper Fajita Bowls

Preparation Time: 10 minutes

Cooking Time: 15 minutes

Servings: 4

Ingredients:

- 4 tbsp. extra-virgin olive oil, divided
- 1 head cauliflower, riced
- 1 lb. (454 g) sirloin steak, cut into ¼-inch-thick strips
- 1 red bell pepper, seeded and sliced
- 1 onion, thinly sliced
- 2 garlic cloves, minced
- 2 limes juice
- 1 tsp. chili powder

Directions:

1. Preheat the air fryer oven to 400°F (205°C).
2. Heat 2 tablespoons of olive oil until it shimmers.
3. Add the cauliflower. Cook, stirring occasionally, until it softens, about 3 minutes. Set aside.
4. Add the remaining 2 tablespoons of oil to the air fryer, and heat it on medium-high until it shimmers.
5. Add the steak and cook, stirring occasionally, until it browns, about 3 minutes. Use a

slotted spoon to remove the steak from the oil in the pan and set it aside.

6. Add the bell pepper and onion to the pan. Cook, stirring occasionally, until they start to brown, about 5 minutes.

7. Add the garlic and cook, stirring constantly, for 30 seconds.

8. Return the beef along with any juices that have been collected and the cauliflower to the pan. Add the lime juice and chili powder. Cook, stirring, until everything is warmed through, 2 to 3 minutes.

Nutrition:

- Calories: 310
- Fat: 18 g
- Protein: 27 g
- Carbs: 13 g
- Sugars: 2 g
- Fiber: 3 g
- Sodium: 93 mg

CHAPTER 14.
POULTRY DINNER RECIPES

121.   Warm Chicken and Spinach Salad

Preparation Time: 10 minutes

Cooking Time: 16-20 minutes

Servings: 4

Ingredients:

- 3 (5 oz.) low-sodium boneless, skinless chicken breasts, cut into 1-inch cubes
- 5 tsp. olive oil
- 1/2 tsp. dried thyme
- 1 medium red onion, sliced
- 1 red bell pepper, sliced
- 1 small zucchini, cut into strips
- 3 tbsp. freshly squeezed lemon juice
- 6 cups fresh baby spinach

Directions:

1. In a huge bowl, blend the chicken with olive oil and thyme. Toss to coat. Transfer to a medium metal bowl and roast for 8 minutes in the air fryer.
2. Add the red onion, red bell pepper, and zucchini. Roast for 8 to 12 more minutes, stirring once during cooking, or until the chicken grasps an inner temperature of 165°F on a meat thermometer.
3. Remove the bowl from the air fryer and stir in the lemon juice.
4. Lay the spinach in a serving bowl and top with the chicken mixture. Toss to combine and serve immediately.

Nutrition:

- Calories: 214
- Fat: 7 g (29% of calories from fat)
- Saturated Fat: 1 g
- Protein: 28 g
- Carbs: 7 g
- Sodium: 116 mg
- Fiber: 2 g

122.   Duo Crisp Chicken Wings

Preparation Time: 10 minutes

Cooking Time: 18 minutes

Servings: 4

Ingredients:

- 12 chicken vignettes
- 1/2 cup chicken broth
- Salt and black pepper to taste
- 1/4 cup melted butter

Directions:

1. Set a metal rack in the air fryer oven and pour broth into it.
2. Place the vignettes on the metal rack, then put on its pressure-cooking lid.
3. Hit the "Pressure Button" and select 8 minutes of cooking time, then press "Start."
4. Once the air fryer oven beeps, do a quick release and remove its lid.
5. Transfer the pressure-cooked vignettes to a plate.
6. Empty the pot and set an air fryer basket in the oven.
7. Toss the vignettes with butter and seasoning.
8. Spread the seasoned vignettes in the air fryer basket.
9. Put on the lid and hit the "Air Fryer Button," then set the time to 10 minutes.
10. Remove the lid and serve.
11. Enjoy!

Nutrition:

- Calories 246
- Total Fat 18.9g
- Saturated Fat 7g
- Cholesterol 115mg
- Sodium 149mg
- Total Carbs: 0 g
- Dietary Fiber: 0 g
- Total Sugars: 0 g
- Protein: 20.2 g

123.   Italian Whole Chicken

Preparation Time: 10 minutes

Cooking Time: 35 minutes

Servings: 4

Ingredients:

- 1 whole chicken
- 2 tbsp. or oil spray of choice
- 1 tsp. garlic powder
- 1 tsp. onion powder
- 1 tsp. paprika
- 1 tsp. Italian seasoning
- 2 tbsp. Montreal steak seasoning
- 1½ cup chicken broth

Directions:

1. Whisk all the seasonings in a bowl and rub it on the chicken.
2. Set a metal rack in the air fryer oven and pour broth into it.
3. Place the chicken on the metal rack, then put on its pressure-cooking lid.
4. Hit the "Pressure Button" and select 25 minutes of cooking time, then press "Start."
5. Once the air fryer oven beeps, do a natural release and remove its lid.
6. Transfer the pressure-cooked chicken to a plate.
7. Empty the pot and set an air fryer basket in the oven.

8. Toss the chicken pieces with oil to coat well.

9. Spread the seasoned chicken in the air fryer basket.

10. Put on the lid and hit the "Air Fryer Button," then set the time to 10 minutes.

11. Remove the lid and serve.

12. Enjoy!

Nutrition:

- Calories: 163
- Total Fat: 10.7 g
- Saturated Fat: 2 g
- Cholesterol: 33 mg
- Sodium: 1439 mg
- Total Carbs: 1.8 g
- Dietary Fiber: 0.3 g
- Total Sugars: 0.8 g
- Protein: 12.6 g

124. Chicken Pot Pie

Preparation Time: 10 minutes

Cooking Time: 17 minutes

Servings: 3

Ingredients:

- 2 tbsp. olive oil
- 1 pound chicken breast cubed
- 1 tbsp. garlic powder
- 1 tbsp. thyme
- 1 tbsp. pepper
- 1 cup chicken broth
- 12 oz. bag frozen mixed vegetables
- 4 large potatoes cubed
- 10 oz. can chicken soup cream
- 1 cup heavy cream

Directions:

1. Hit the "Sauté Button" on the air fryer oven and add chicken and olive oil.

2. Saute chicken for 5 minutes, then stirs in spices.

3. Pour in the broth along with vegetables and cream of chicken soup.

4. Put on the pressure-cooking lid and seal it.

5. Hit the "Pressure Button" and select 10 minutes of cooking time, then press "Start."

6. Once the air fryer oven beeps, do a quick release and remove its lid.

7. Remove the lid and stir in cream.

8. Hit "Sauté Button" and cook for 2 minutes.

9. Enjoy!

Nutrition:

- Calories 568
- Total Fat 31.1 g
- Saturated Fat: 9.1 g
- Cholesterol: 95 mg
- Sodium: 1111 mg
- Total Carbs: 50.8 g
- Dietary Fiber: 3.9 g
- Total Sugars: 18.8 g
- Protein: 23.4 g

125.　　Chicken Casserole

Preparation Time: 10 minutes

Cooking Time: 9 minutes

Servings: 4

Ingredients:

- 12 oz. bag egg noodles
- 1/2 large onion
- 1/2 cup chopped carrots
- 1/4 cup frozen peas
- 1/4 cup frozen broccoli pieces
- 2 stalks celery chopped
- 5 cups chicken broth
- 1 tsp. garlic powder
- Salt and pepper to taste
- 1 cup cheddar cheese, shredded
- 1 package French's onions
- 1/4 cup sour cream
- 1 can chicken cream and mushroom soup

Directions:

1. Add chicken broth, black pepper, salt, garlic powder, vegetables, and egg noodles to the air fryer oven.
2. Please put on the pressure-cooking lid and seal it.
3. Hit the "Pressure Button" and select 4 minutes of cooking time, then press "Start."
4. Once the air fryer oven beeps, do a quick release and remove its lid.
5. Stir in cheese, 1/3 of French's onions, a can of soup, and sour cream.
6. Mix well and spread the remaining onion on top.
7. Put on the air fryer lid and seal it.
8. Hit the "Air Fryer Button" and select 5 minutes of cooking time, then press "Start."
9. Once the Air Fryer oven beeps, remove its lid.
10. Serve.

Nutrition:

- Calories: 494
- Total Fat: 19.1 g
- Saturated Fat: 9.6 g
- Cholesterol: 142 mg
- Sodium: 1233 mg
- Total Carbs: 29 g
- Dietary Fiber: 2.6 g
- Total Sugars: 3.7 g
- Protein: 48.9 g

126.　　Ranch Chicken Wings

Preparation Time: 10 minutes

Cooking Time: 35 minutes

Servings: 3

Ingredients:

- 12 chicken wings
- 1 tbsp. olive oil

- 1 cup chicken broth
- 1/4 cup butter
- 1/2 cup red hot sauce
- 1/4 tsp. Worcestershire sauce
- 1 tbsp. white vinegar
- 1/4 tsp. cayenne pepper
- 1/8 tsp. garlic powder
- Seasoned salt to taste
- Black pepper
- Ranch dressing for dipping
- Celery to garnish

Directions:

1. Set the air fryer basket in the air fryer oven and pour the broth in it.
2. Spread the chicken wings in the basket and put on the pressure-cooking lid.
3. Hit the "Pressure Button" and select 10 minutes of cooking time, then press "Start."
4. Meanwhile, for the sauce preparation, add butter, vinegar, cayenne pepper, garlic powder, Worcestershire sauce, and spicy sauce in a small saucepan.
5. Stir and cook this sauce for 5 minutes on medium heat until it thickens.
6. Once the air fryer oven beeps, do a quick release and remove its lid.
7. Remove the wings and empty the air fryer oven Duo.
8. Toss the wings with oil, salt, and black pepper.

9. Set the air fryer basket in the oven and arrange the wings in it.
10. Put on the lid and seal it.
11. Hit the "Air Fryer Button" and select 20 minutes of cooking time, then press "Start."
12. Once the air fryer oven beeps, remove its lid.
13. Transfer the wings to the sauce and mix well.
14. Serve.

Nutrition:

- Calories: 414
- Total Fat: 31.6 g
- Saturated Fat: 11 g
- Cholesterol: 98 mg
- Sodium: 568 mg
- Total Carbs: 11.2 g
- Dietary Fiber: 0.3 g
- Total Sugars: 0.2 g
- Protein: 20.4 g

127. Chicken Mac and Cheese

Preparation Time: 10 minutes

Cooking Time: 9 minutes

Servings: 4

Ingredients:

- 2 ½ cups macaroni
- 2 cups chicken stock
- 1 cup cooked chicken, shredded

- 1 ¼ cup heavy cream
- 8 tbsp. butter
- 1 bag Ritz crackers

Directions:

1. Add chicken stock, heavy cream, chicken, 4 tablespoons butter, and macaroni to the air fryer oven Duo.
2. Put on the pressure-cooking lid and seal it.
3. Hit the "Pressure Button" and select 4 minutes of cooking time, then press "Start."
4. Crush the crackers and mix them well with 4 tablespoons melted butter.
5. Once the air fryer oven beeps, do a quick release and remove its lid.
6. Put on the lid and seal it.
7. Hit the "Air Fryer Button" and select 5 minutes of cooking time, then press "Start."
8. Once the air fryer oven beeps, remove its lid.
9. Serve.

Nutrition:

- Calories: 611
- Total Fat: 43.6 g
- Saturated Fat: 26.8 g
- Cholesterol: 147 mg
- Sodium: 739 mg
- Total Carbs: 29.5 g
- Dietary Fiber: 1.2 g
- Total Sugars: 1.7 g
- Protein: 25.4 g

128. Broccoli Chicken Casserole

Preparation Time: 10 minutes

Cooking Time: 22 minutes

Servings: 4

Ingredients:

- 1 ½ lb. chicken, cubed
- 2 tsp. chopped garlic
- 2 tbsp. butter
- 1 ½ cup chicken broth
- 1 ½ cup long-grain rice
- 1 (10.75 oz.) can chicken soup cream
- 2 cups broccoli florets
- 1 cup crushed Ritz cracker
- 2 tbsp. melted butter
- 2 cups shredded cheddar cheese
- 1 cup water

Directions:

1. Swell 1 cup water into the air fryer oven Duo and place a basket in it.
2. Place the broccoli in the basket evenly.
3. Put on the pressure-cooking lid and seal it.
4. Hit the "Pressure Button" and select 1 minute of cooking time, then press "Start."
5. Once the air fryer oven beeps, do a quick release and remove its lid.
6. Remove the broccoli and empty the air fryer oven Duo.

7. Hit the "Sauté Button," then add 2 tablespoons butter.

8. Toss in chicken and stir cook for 5 minutes, then add garlic and saute for 30 seconds.

9. Stir in rice, chicken broth, and cream of chicken soup.

10. Put on the pressure-cooking lid and seal it.

11. Hit the "Pressure Button" and select 12 minutes of cooking time, then press "Start."

12. Once the air fryer oven beeps, do a quick release and remove its lid.

13. Add cheese and broccoli, then mix well gently.

14. Toss the cracker with 2 tablespoons butter in a bowl and spread over the pot's chicken.

15. Put on the lid and seal it.

16. Hit the "Air Fryer Button" and select 4 minutes of cooking time, then press "Start."

17. Once the air fryer oven beeps, remove its lid.

18. Serve.

Nutrition:
- Calories: 609
- Total Fat: 24.4 g
- Saturated: Fat 12.6 g
- Cholesterol: 142 mg
- Sodium: 924mg
- Total Carbs: 45.5 g
- Dietary Fiber: 1.4 g
- Total Sugars: 1.6 g
- Protein: 49.2 g

129. Chicken Tikka Kebab

Preparation Time: 10 minutes

Cooking Time: 17 minutes

Servings: 4

Ingredients:

- 1 lb. chicken thighs boneless skinless, cubed
- 1 tbsp. oil
- 1/2 cup red onion, cubed
- 1/2 cup green bell pepper, cubed
- 1/2 cup red bell pepper, cubed
- Lime wedges and Onion rounds to garnish

For marinade:

- 1/2 cup yogurt Greek
- 3/4 tbsp. ginger, grated
- 3/4 tbsp. garlic, minced
- 1 tbsp. lime juice
- 2 tsp. red chili powder mild
- 1/2 tsp. ground turmeric
- 1 tsp. garam masala
- 1 tsp. coriander powder
- 1/2 tbsp. dried fenugreek leaves
- 1 tsp. salt

Directions:

1. Preparation of the marinade by mixing yogurt with all its ingredients in a bowl.
2. Fold in chicken, then mix well to coat and refrigerate for 8 hours.
3. Add bell pepper, onions, and oil to the marinade and mix well.
4. Yarn the chicken, peppers, and onions on the skewers.
5. Set the air fryer basket in the oven Duo.
6. Put on the lid and seal it.
7. Hit the "Air Fryer Button" and select 10 minutes of cooking time, then press "Start."
8. Once the air fryer oven beeps, and remove its lid.
9. Flip the skewers and continue air frying for 7 minutes.
10. Serve.

Nutrition:

- Calories: 241
- Total Fat: 14.2 g
- Saturated Fat: 3.8 g
- Cholesterol: 92 mg
- Sodium: 695 mg
- Total Carbs: 8.5 g
- Dietary Fiber: 1.6 g
- Total Sugars: 3.9 g
- Protein: 21.8 g

130. Bacon-Wrapped Chicken

Preparation Time: 10 minutes

Cooking Time: 24 minutes

Servings: 4

Ingredients:

- 1/4 cup maple syrup
- 1 tsp. ground black pepper
- 1 tsp. Dijon mustard
- 1/4 tsp. garlic powder
- 1/8 tsp. kosher salt
- 4 (6 oz.) skinless, boneless chicken breasts
- 8 slices bacon

Directions:

1. Whisk maple syrup with salt, garlic powder, mustard, and black pepper in a small bowl.
2. Rub the chicken with salt and black pepper, and wrap each chicken breast with 2 slices of bacon.
3. Place the wrapped chicken in the Air fryer oven baking pan.
4. Brush the wrapped chicken with maple syrup mixture.
5. Put on the lid and seal it.
6. Hit the "Bake Button" and select 20 cooking times, then press "Start."
7. Once the function is completed, switch the pot to "Broil" mode and cook for 4 minutes.
8. Serve.

Nutrition:

- Calories: 441
- Total Fat: 18.3 g
- Saturated Fat: 5.2 g
- Cholesterol: 141 mg
- Sodium: 1081 mg
- Total Carbs: 14 g
- Dietary Fiber: 0.1 g
- Total Sugars: 11.8 g
- Protein: 53.6 g

131. Creamy Chicken Thighs

Preparation Time: 10 minutes

Cooking Time: 30 minutes

Servings: 2

Ingredients:

- 1 tbsp. olive oil
- 6 chicken thighs, bone-in, skin-on
- Salt
- Freshly ground black pepper
- 3/4 cup low-sodium chicken broth
- 1/2 cup heavy cream
- 1/2 cup sun-dried tomatoes, chopped
- 1/4 cup Parmesan, grated
- Freshly torn basil to serve

Directions:

1. Hit the "Sauté Button" on the Air fryer oven and add oil to heat.
2. Stir in chicken, salt, and black pepper, then sear for 5 minutes per side.
3. Add broth, cream, parmesan, and tomatoes.
4. Put on the Air Fryer lid and seal it.
5. Hit the "Bake Button" and select 20 minutes of cooking time, then press "Start."
6. Once the Air Fryer oven beeps, remove its lid.
7. Garnish with basil and serve.

Nutrition:

- Calories 454
- Total Fat 37.8g
- Saturated Fat 14.4g
- Cholesterol 169mg
- Sodium: 181 mg
- Total Carbs: 2.8 g
- Dietary Fiber: 0.7 g
- Total Sugars: 0.7 g
- Protein: 26.9 g

132. Air Fryer Teriyaki Hen Drumsticks

Preparation Time: 30 minutes

Cooking Time: 20 minutes

Servings: 4

Ingredients:

- 6 poultry drumsticks
- 1 mug teriyaki sauce

Directions:

1. Mix drumsticks with teriyaki sauce in a zip-lock bag. Let the sauce rest for half an hour.
2. Preheat your air fryer to 360°F.
3. Abode the drumsticks in one layer in the air fryer basket and cook for 20 minutes. Shake the basket pair times through food preparation.
4. Garnish with sesame seeds and sliced onions

Nutrition:

- Calories: 163
- Carbs: 7 g
- Protein: 16 g
- Fat: 7 g

CHAPTER 15. APPETIZER AND SIDES RECIPES

82.   Cucumber Tomato Avocado Salad

Preparation time: 10 minutes

Cooking time: 0 minutes

Servings: 4

Ingredients:

- 1 cup cherry tomatoes, halved
- 1 large cucumber, chopped
- 1 small red onion, thinly sliced
- 1 avocado, diced
- 2 tbsp. chopped fresh dill
- 2 tbsp. extra-virgin olive oil
- Juice of 1 lemon
- 1/4 tsp. salt
- 1/4 tsp. freshly ground black pepper

Directions:

1. In a large mixing bowl, combine the tomatoes, cucumber, onion, avocado, and dill.
2. In a small bowl, combine the oil, lemon juice, salt, and pepper, and mix well.
3. Drizzle the dressing over the vegetables and toss to combine. Serve.

Nutrition:

- Calories: 151
- Carbohydrates: 11 g
- Protein: 2 g
- Fat: 12 g
- Sugars: 4 g
- Fiber: 4 g
- Sodium: 128 mg

83.   Cabbage and Carrot Slaw

Preparation time: 15 minutes

Cooking time: 0 minutes

Servings: 2

Ingredients:

- 2 cups finely chopped green cabbage
- 2 cups finely chopped red cabbage
- 2 cups grated carrots
- 3 scallions, both white and green parts, sliced
- 2 tbsp. extra-virgin olive oil
- 2 tbsp. rice vinegar
- 1 tsp. honey
- 1 garlic clove, minced
- 1/4 tsp. salt

Directions:

1. In a large bowl, toss together the green and red cabbage, carrots, and scallions.

2. In a small bowl, whisk together the oil, vinegar, honey, garlic, and salt.

3. Pour the dressing over the veggies and mix to thoroughly combine.

4. Serve immediately, or cover and chill for several hours before serving.

Nutrition:

- Calories: 80
- Carbohydrates: 10 g
- Protein: 1 g
- Fat: 5 g
- Sugars: 6 g
- Fiber: 3 g
- Sodium: 126 mg

84.   Blackberry Goat Cheese Salad

Preparation time: 15 minutes

Cooking time: 20 minutes

Servings: 4

Ingredients:

Vinaigrette:

- 1-pint blackberries
- 2 tbsp. red wine vinegar
- 1 tbsp. honey
- 3 tbsp. extra-virgin olive oil
- 1/4 tsp. salt
- Freshly ground black pepper, to taste

Salad:

- 1 sweet potato, cubed
- 1 tsp. extra-virgin olive oil
- 8 cups salad greens (baby spinach, spicy greens, romaine)
- 1/2 red onion, sliced
- 1/4 cup crumbled goat cheese

Make the vinaigrette:

1. In a blender jar, combine the blackberries, vinegar, honey, oil, salt, and pepper, and process until smooth. Set aside.

Make the salad:

2. Preheat the oven to 425°F (220°C). Line a baking sheet with parchment paper.

3. In a medium mixing bowl, toss the sweet potato with olive oil. Transfer to the prepared baking sheet and roast for 20 minutes, stirring once halfway through, until tender. Remove and cool for a few minutes.

4. In a large bowl, toss the greens with the red onion and cooled sweet potato, and

drizzle with the vinaigrette. Serve topped with 1 tbsp. goat cheese per serving.

Nutrition:

- Calories: 196
- Carbohydrates: 21 g
- Protein: 3 g
- Fat: 12 g
- Sugars: 10 g
- Fiber: 6 g
- Sodium: 184 mg

85. Garlic and Basil Three Bean Salad

Preparation time: 10 minutes

Cooking time: 0 minutes

Servings: 2

Ingredients:

- 1 (15 oz./425 g) can low-sodium chickpeas, drained and rinsed
- 1 (15 oz./425 g) can low-sodium kidney beans, drained and rinsed
- 1 (15 oz./425 g) can low-sodium white beans, drained and rinsed
- 1 red bell pepper, seeded and finely chopped
- ¼ cup chopped scallions, both white and green parts
- ¼ cup finely chopped fresh basil
- 3 garlic cloves, minced
- 2 tbsp. extra-virgin olive oil
- 1 tbsp. red wine vinegar
- 1 tsp. Dijon mustard
- ¼ tsp. freshly ground black pepper

Directions:

1. In a large mixing bowl, combine the chickpeas, kidney beans, white beans, bell pepper, scallions, basil, and garlic. Toss gently to combine.
2. In a small bowl, combine the olive oil, vinegar, mustard, and pepper. Toss with the salad.
3. Cover and refrigerate for an hour before serving, to allow the flavors to mix.

Nutrition:

- Calories: 193
- Carbohydrates: 29 g
- Protein: 10 g
- Fat: 5 g
- Sugars: 3 g
- Fiber: 8 g
- Sodium: 246 mg

86. Rainbow Black Bean Salad

Preparation time: 15 minutes

Cooking time: 0 minutes

Servings: 3

Ingredients:

- 1 (15 oz./425 g) can low-sodium black beans, drained and rinsed
- 1 avocado, diced
- 2 Tomatoes halved
- 1 cup chopped baby spinach
- 1/2 cup finely chopped red bell pepper
- 1/4 cup finely chopped jicama
- 1/2 cup chopped scallions, both white and green parts
- 1/4 cup chopped fresh cilantro
- 2 tbsp. freshly squeezed lime juice
- 1 tbsp. extra-virgin olive oil
- 2 garlic cloves, minced
- 1 tsp. honey
- 1/4 tsp. salt
- 1/4 tsp. freshly ground black pepper

Directions:

1. In a large bowl, combine the black beans, avocado, tomatoes, spinach, bell pepper, jicama, scallions, and cilantro.
2. In a small bowl, mix the lime juice, oil, garlic, honey, salt, and pepper. Add to the salad and toss.

Nutrition:

- Calories: 169
- Carbohydrates: 22 g

- Protein: 6 g
- Fat: 7 g
- Sugars: 3 g
- Fiber: 9 g
- Sodium: 235 mg

87. Squash and Barley Salad

Preparation time: 20 minutes

Cooking time: 40 minutes

Servings: 2

Ingredients:

- 1 small butternut squash
- 3 tsp. + 2 tbsp. extra-virgin olive oil, divided
- 2 cups broccoli florets
- 1 cup pearl barley
- 1 cup toasted chopped walnuts
- 2 cups baby kale
- 1/2 red onion, sliced
- 2 tbsp. balsamic vinegar
- 2 garlic cloves, minced
- 1/2 tsp. salt
- 1/4 tsp. freshly ground black pepper
- 2 cups of water

Directions:

1. Preheat the oven to 400°F (205°C). Line a baking sheet with parchment paper.

2. Peel and seed the squash, and cut it into dice. In a large bowl, toss the squash with 2 tsp. olive oil. Transfer to the prepared baking sheet and roast for 20 minutes.

3. While the squash is roasting, toss the broccoli in the same bowl with 1 tsp. olive oil. After 20 minutes, flip the squash and

   push it to one side of the baking sheet. Add the broccoli to the other side and continue to roast for 20 more minutes until tender.

4. While the veggies are roasting, in a medium pot, cover the barley with water. Bring to a boil, then reduce the heat, cover, and simmer for 30 minutes until tender. Drain and rinse.

5. Transfer the barley to a large bowl, and toss with the cooked squash and broccoli, walnuts, kale, and onion.

6. In a small bowl, mix the remaining 2 tbsp. olive oil, balsamic vinegar, garlic, salt, and pepper. Toss the salad with the dressing and serve.

Nutrition:

- Calories: 275
- Carbohydrates: 32 g
- Protein: 6 g
- Fat: 15 g
- Sugars: 3 g
- Fiber: 7 g

- Sodium: 144 mg

88. Winter Chicken Salad with Citrus

Preparation time: 10 minutes

Cooking time: 0 minutes

Servings: 4

Ingredients:

- 4 cups baby spinach
- 2 tbsp. extra-virgin olive oil
- 1 tbsp. freshly squeezed lemon juice
- 1/8 tsp. salt
- Freshly ground black pepper, to taste
- 2 cups chopped cooked chicken
- 2 mandarin oranges, peeled and segmented
- 1/2 peeled grapefruit, segmented
- 1/4 cup sliced almonds

Directions:

1. In a large mixing bowl, toss the spinach with olive oil, lemon juice, salt, and pepper.
2. Add the chicken, mandarin oranges, grapefruit, and almonds to the bowl. Toss gently.

Nutrition:

- Calories: 249

- Carbohydrates: 11 g
- Protein: 24 g
- Fat: 12 g
- Sugars: 7 g
- Fiber: 3 g
- Sodium: 135 mg

89.   Blueberry Chicken Salad

Preparation time: 10 minutes

Cooking time: 0 minutes

Servings: 4

Ingredients:

- 2 cups chopped cooked chicken
- 1 cup fresh blueberries
- 1/4 cup finely chopped almonds
- 1 celery stalk, finely chopped
- 1/4 cup finely chopped red onion
- 1 tbsp. chopped fresh basil
- 1 tbsp. chopped fresh cilantro
- 1/2 cup plain, nonfat Greek yogurt or vegan mayonnaise
- 1/4 tsp. salt
- 1/4 tsp. freshly ground black pepper
- 8 cups salad greens (baby spinach, spicy greens, romaine)

Directions:

1. In a large mixing bowl, combine the chicken, blueberries, almonds, celery, onion, basil, and cilantro. Toss gently to mix.
2. In a small bowl, combine the yogurt, salt, and pepper. Add to the chicken salad and stir to combine.
3. Arrange 2 cups of salad greens on each of 4 plates and divide the chicken salad among the plates to serve.

Nutrition:

- Calories: 207
- Carbohydrates: 11 g
- Protein: 28 g
- Fat: 6 g
- Sugars: 6 g
- Fiber: 3 g
- Sodium: 235 mg

90.   Quinoa, Salmon, and Avocado Salad

Preparation time: 15 minutes

Cooking time: 20 minutes

Servings: 4

Ingredients:

- 1/2 cup quinoa
- 1 cup water

- 4 (4 oz./113 g) salmon fillets
- 1 lb. (454 g) asparagus, trimmed
- 1 tsp. + 2 tbsp. extra-virgin olive oil
- 1/2 tsp. salt, divided
- 1/2 tsp. freshly ground black pepper, divided
- 1/4 tsp. red pepper flakes
- 1 avocado, chopped
- 1/4 cup chopped scallions, both white and green parts
- 1/4 cup chopped fresh cilantro
- 1 tbsp. minced fresh oregano
- Juice of 1 lime

Directions:

1. In a small pot, combine the quinoa and water, and bring to a boil over medium-high heat. Cover, reduce the heat, and simmer for 15 minutes.
2. Preheat the oven to 425°F (220°C). Line a large baking sheet with parchment paper.
3. Arrange the salmon on one side of the prepared baking sheet. Toss the asparagus with 1 tsp. olive oil, and arrange it on the other side of the baking sheet. Season the salmon and asparagus with 1/4 tsp. salt, 1/4 tsp. pepper, and red pepper flakes. Roast for 12 minutes until browned and cooked through.
4. While the fish and asparagus are cooking, in a large mixing bowl, gently toss the cooked quinoa, avocado, scallions, cilantro, and oregano. Add the remaining 2 tbsp. olive oil and the lime juice, and season with the remaining 1/4 tsp. salt and 1/4 tsp. pepper.
5. Break the salmon into pieces, removing the skin and any bones, and chop the asparagus into bite-sized pieces. Fold into the quinoa and serve warm or at room temperature.

Nutrition:

- Calories: 397
- Carbohydrates: 23 g
- Protein: 29 g
- Fat: 22 g
- Sugars: 3 g
- Fiber: 8 g
- Sodium: 292 mg

91. Sautéed Spinach and Cherry Tomatoes

Preparation time: 5 minutes

Cooking time: 10 minutes

Servings: 4

Ingredients:

- 1 tbsp. extra-virgin olive oil
- 1 cup cherry tomatoes, halved
- 3 spinach bunches, trimmed

- 2 garlic cloves, minced
- 1/4 tsp. salt

Directions:

1. In a large skillet, heat the oil over medium heat.
2. Add the tomatoes, and cook until the skins begin to blister and split, about 2 minutes.
3. Add the spinach in batches, waiting for each batch to wilt slightly before adding the next batch. Stir continuously for 3 to 4 minutes until the spinach is tender.
4. Add the garlic to the skillet, and toss until fragrant, about 30 seconds.
5. Drain the excess liquid from the pan. Add the salt. Stir well and serve.

Nutrition:

- Calories: 52
- Carbohydrates: 4 g
- Protein: 2 g
- Fat: 4 g
- Sugars: 1 g
- Fiber: 2 g
- Sodium: 183 mg

92.   Garlicky Cabbage and Collard Greens

Preparation time: 10 minutes

Cooking time: 10 minutes

Servings: 4

Ingredients:

- 2 tbsp. extra-virgin olive oil
- 1 collard greens bunch, stemmed and thinly sliced
- 1/2 small green cabbage, thinly sliced
- 6 garlic cloves, minced
- 1 tbsp. low-sodium gluten-free soy sauce or tamari

Directions:

1. In a large skillet, heat the oil over medium-high heat.
2. Add the collards to the pan, stirring to coat with oil. Sauté for 1 to 2 minutes until the greens begin to wilt.
3. Add the cabbage and stir to coat. Cover and reduce the heat to medium-low. Continue to cook for 5 to 7 minutes, stirring once or twice, until the greens are tender.
4. Add the garlic and soy sauce and stir to incorporate. Cook until just fragrant, about 30 seconds longer. Serve warm and enjoy!

Nutrition:

- Calories: 72
- Carbohydrates: 6 g
- Protein: 3 g

- Fat: 4 g
- Sugars: 0 g
- Fiber: 3 g
- Sodium: 129 mg

93.   Roasted Lemon and Garlic Broccoli

Preparation time: 10 minutes

Cooking time: 25 minutes

Servings: 3

Ingredients:

- 2 large broccoli heads, cut into florets
- 3 garlic cloves, minced
- 2 tbsp. extra-virgin olive oil
- 1/4 tsp. salt
- 1/4 tsp. freshly ground black pepper
- 2 tbsp. freshly squeezed lemon juice

Directions:

1. Preheat the oven to 425°F (220°C).
2. On a rimmed baking sheet, toss the broccoli, garlic, and olive oil. Season with salt and pepper.
3. Roast, tossing occasionally, for 25 to 30 minutes until tender and browned. Season with lemon juice and serve.

Nutrition:

- Calories: 30
- Carbohydrates: 3 g
- Protein: 1 g
- Fat: 2 g
- Sugars: 1 g
- Fiber: 1 g
- Sodium: 84 mg

94.   Cauli-Broccoli Tots

Preparation time: 10 minutes

Cooking time: 20 minutes

Servings: 4

Ingredients:

- 1 cup chopped broccoli florets and stems
- 1 cup chopped cauliflower florets and stems
- 1/4 cup diced onion
- 1 large egg
- 1/4 cup whole-wheat breadcrumbs
- 1/4 cup crumbled feta cheese
- 1/2 tsp. salt
- 1/4 tsp. freshly ground black pepper

Directions:

1. Preheat the oven to 400°F (205°C). Line a baking sheet with parchment paper.
2. In a food processor, combine the broccoli, cauliflower, and onion, and pulse until

chopped well but still slightly chunky. Or if you don't have a food processor, chop everything on a large cutting board until you have very small pieces. Transfer to a large mixing bowl.

3. Add the egg, breadcrumbs, cheese, salt, and pepper.

4. Using your hands, shape small balls, a little smaller than a tbsp., and carefully place those on the prepared baking sheet.

5. Bake for 10 minutes, flip carefully, and continue to bake for 10 additional minutes until browned and crisp.

Nutrition:

- Calories: 90
- Carbohydrates: 9 g
- Protein: 5 g
- Fat: 4 g
- Sugars: 2 g
- Fiber: 2 g
- Sodium: 424 mg

95.   Spicy Roasted Cauliflower with Lime

Preparation time: 5 minutes

Cooking time: 10 minutes

Servings: 4

Ingredients:

- 1 cauliflower head, broken into small florets
- 2 tbsp. extra-virgin olive oil
- 1/2 tsp. ground chipotle chili powder
- 1/2 tsp. salt
- Juice of 1 lime

Directions:

1. Preheat the oven to 450°F (235°C). Line a rimmed baking sheet with parchment paper.

2. In a large mixing bowl, toss the cauliflower with olive oil, chipotle chili powder, and salt. Arrange in a single layer on the prepared baking sheet.

3. Roast for 15 minutes, flip and continue to roast for 15 more minutes until well-browned and tender.

4. Sprinkle with the lime juice, adjust the salt as needed, and serve.

Nutrition:

- Calories: 99
- Carbohydrates: 8 g
- Protein: 3 g
- Fat: 7 g
- Sugars: 3 g
- Fiber: 3 g
- Sodium: 284 mg

96.   Roasted Delicata Squash

Preparation time: 10 minutes

Cooking time: 20 minutes

Servings: 4

Ingredients:

- 1 (1 to 1 1/2 lb./454 to 680 g) delicata squash, halved, seeded, cut into 1/2-inch-thick strips
- 1 tbsp. extra-virgin olive oil
- 1/2 tsp. dried thyme
- 1/4 tsp. salt
- 1/4 tsp. freshly ground black pepper

Directions:

1. Preheat the oven to 400°F (205°C). Line a baking sheet with parchment paper.
2. In a large mixing bowl, toss the squash strips with olive oil, thyme, salt, and pepper. Arrange on the prepared baking sheet in a single layer.
3. Roast for 10 minutes, flip and continue to roast for 10 more minutes until tender and lightly browned.

Nutrition:

- Calories: 79
- Carbohydrates: 12 g
- Protein: 1 g
- Fat: 4 g
- Sugars: 3 g
- Fiber: 2 g
- Sodium: 123 mg

97.   Roasted Asparagus, Onions, and Red Peppers

Preparation time: 5 minutes

Cooking time: 20 minutes

Servings: 4

Ingredients:

- 1 lb. (454 g) asparagus, woody ends trimmed, cut into 2-inch segments
- 1 small onion, quartered
- 2 red bell peppers, seeded, cut into 1-inch pieces
- 2 tbsp. Easy Italian Dressing

Directions:

1. Preheat the oven to 400°F (205°C). Line a baking sheet with parchment paper.
2. In a large mixing bowl, toss the asparagus, onion, and peppers with the dressing. Transfer to the prepared baking sheet.

3. Roast for 10 minutes, then, using a spatula, flip the vegetables. Roast for 5 to 10 more minutes until the vegetables are tender.

4. Stir well and serve.

Nutrition:

- Calories: 93
- Carbohydrates: 11 g
- Protein: 3 g
- Fat: 5 g
- Sugars: 6 g
- Fiber: 4 g
- Sodium: 32 mg

98.   Green Bean Casserole

Preparation time: 10 minutes

Cooking time: 30 minutes

Servings: 2

Ingredients:

- 1 lb. (454 g) green beans, trimmed, cut into bite-size pieces
- 3 tbsp. extra-virgin olive oil, divided
- 8 oz. (227 g) brown mushrooms, diced
- 3 garlic cloves, minced
- 1 1/2 tbsp. whole-wheat flour
- 1 cup low-sodium vegetable broth
- 1 cup unsweetened plain almond milk
- 1/4 cup almond flour
- 2 tbsp. dried minced onion

Directions:

1. Preheat the oven to 400°F (205°C).

2. Bring a large pot of water to a boil. Boil the green beans for 3 to 5 minutes until just barely tender but still bright green. Drain and set aside.

3. In a medium skillet, heat 2 tbsp. oil over medium-high heat. Add the mushrooms and stir. Cook for 3 to 5 minutes until the mushrooms brown and release their liquid. Add the garlic and stir until just fragrant, about 30 seconds.

4. Add the whole-wheat flour and stir well to combine. Add the broth and simmer for 1 minute.

5. Reduce the heat to medium-low and add the almond milk. Return to a simmer and cook for 5 to 7 minutes until the mixture thickens.

6. Remove from the heat. Stir in the green beans and transfer them to a baking dish.

7. In a small bowl, mix the almond flour, dried minced onion, and remaining 1 tbsp. olive oil, and stir until combined and crumbly. Crumble over the beans.

8. Bake for 15 to 20 minutes until the liquids are bubbling and the top is browned.

Nutrition:

- Calories: 97
- Carbohydrates: 7 g
- Protein: 2 g
- Fat: 7 g
- Sugars: 2 g
- Fiber: 2 g
- Sodium: 57 mg

99. Tomato, Peach, and Strawberry Salad

Preparation time: 15 minutes

Cooking time: 0 minutes

Servings: 3

Ingredients:

- 6 cups mixed spring greens
- 4 large ripe plum tomatoes, thinly sliced
- 4 large ripe peaches, pitted and thinly sliced
- 12 ripe strawberries, thinly sliced
- 1/2 Vidalia onion, thinly sliced
- 2 tbsp. white balsamic vinegar
- 2 tbsp. extra-virgin olive oil
- Freshly ground black pepper, to taste

Directions:

1. Put the greens in a large salad bowl, and layer the tomatoes, peaches, strawberries, and onion on top.
2. Dress with the vinegar and oil, toss together, and season with pepper.

Nutrition:

- Calories: 127
- Carbohydrates: 19 g
- Protein: 4 g
- Fat: 5 g
- Sugars: 13 g
- Fiber: 5 g
- Sodium: 30 mg

100. Raw Corn Salad with Black-Eyed Peas

Preparation time: 15 minutes

Cooking time: 0 minutes

Servings: 4

Ingredients:

- 2 ears fresh corn, kernels cut off
- 2 cups cooked black-eyed peas
- 1 green bell pepper, chopped
- 1/2 red onion, chopped
- 2 celery stalks, finely chopped

- 1/2-pint cherry tomatoes halved
- 3 tbsp. white balsamic vinegar
- 2 tbsp. extra-virgin olive oil
- 1 garlic clove, minced
- 1/4 tsp. smoked paprika
- 1/4 tsp. ground cumin
- 1/4 tsp. red pepper flakes

Directions:

1. In a large salad bowl, combine the corn, black-eyed peas, bell pepper, onion, celery, and tomatoes.
2. In a small bowl, to make the dressing, whisk the vinegar, olive oil, garlic, and paprika, cumin, and red pepper flakes together.
3. Pour the dressing over the salad, and toss gently to coat. Serve and enjoy.

Nutrition:

- Calories: 123
- Carbohydrates: 18 g
- Protein: 5 g
- Fat: 5 g
- Sugars: 3 g
- Fiber: 4 g
- Sodium: 24 mg

101. Young Kale and Cabbage Salad

Preparation time: 15 minutes

Cooking time: 0 minutes

Servings: 3

Ingredients:

- 2 bunches of baby kale, thinly sliced
- 1/2 head green savoy cabbage, cored and thinly sliced
- 1/4 cup apple cider vinegar
- Juice of 1 lemon
- 1 tsp. ground cumin
- 1/4 tsp. smoked paprika
- 1 medium red bell pepper, thinly sliced
- 1 cup toasted peanuts
- 1 garlic clove, thinly sliced

Directions:

1. In a large salad bowl, toss the kale and cabbage together.
2. In a small bowl, to make the dressing, whisk the vinegar, lemon juice, cumin, and paprika together.
3. Pour the dressing over the greens, and gently massage with your hands.
4. Add the pepper, peanuts, and garlic, and toss to combine.

Nutrition:

- Calories: 199
- Carbohydrates: 17 g
- Protein: 10 g

- Fat: 12 g
- Sugars: 4 g
- Fiber: 5 g
- Sodium: 46 mg

153.　Garlic Kale Chips

Preparation Time: 6−7 minutes

Cooking Time: 5 minutes

Servings: 2

Ingredients:

- 1 tbsp. yeast flakes
- Sea salt to taste
- 4 cups packed kale
- 2 tbsp. olive oil
- 1 tsp. garlic, minced
- 1/2 cup ranch seasoning pieces

Directions:

1. In a bowl, place the oil, kale, garlic, and ranch seasoning pieces. Add the yeast and mix well. Dump the coated kale into an air fryer basket and cook at 375°F for 5 minutes.
2. Shake after 3 minutes and serve.

Nutrition:

- Calories: 50
- Total Fat: 1.9 g
- Carbs: 10 g
- Protein: 46 g

154.　Garlic Salmon Balls

Preparation Time: 6−7 minutes

Cooking Time: 10 minutes

- **Servings:** 2

Ingredients:

- 6 oz. tinned salmon
- 1 large egg
- 3 tbsp. olive oil
- 5 tbsp. wheat germ
- 1/2 tsp. garlic powder
- 1 tbsp. dill, fresh, chopped
- 4 tbsp. spring onion, diced
- 4 tbsp. celery, diced

Directions:

1. Preheat your air fryer to 370°F. In a large bowl, mix the salmon, egg, celery, onion, dill, and garlic.
2. Shape the mixture into golf ball size balls and roll them in the wheat germ. In a minor pan, warm olive oil over medium-low heat. Add the salmon balls and slowly flatten them. Handover them to your air fryer and cook for 10 minutes.

Nutrition:

- Calories: 219
- Total Fat: 7.7 g

- Carbs: 14.8 g
- Protein: 23.1 g

155.   Onion Rings

Preparation Time: 7 minutes

Cooking Time: 10 minutes

Servings: 3

Ingredients:

- 1 onion, cut into slices, then separate into rings
- 1 ½ cup almond flour
- 3/4 cup pork rinds
- 1 cup milk
- 1 egg
- 1 tbsp. baking powder
- 1/2 tsp. salt

Directions:

1. Preheat your air fryer for 10 minutes. Cut onion into slices, then separate into rings. In a container, supplement the flour, baking powder, and salt.
2. Whisk the eggs and the milk, then combines with flour. Gently dip the floured onion rings into the batter to coat them.
3. Spread the pork rinds on a plate and dredge the rings in the crumbs. Abode the onion rings in your air fryer and cook for 10 minutes at 360°F.

Nutrition:

- Calories: 304
- Total Fat: 18g
- Carbs: 31g
- Protein: 38g

156.   Crispy Eggplant Fries

Preparation Time: 7 minutes

Cooking Time: 12 minutes

Servings: 3

Ingredients:

- 2 eggplants
- 1/4 cup olive oil
- 1/4 cup almond flour
- 1/2 cup water

Directions:

1. Preheat your air fryer to 390°F. Cut the eggplants into ½-inch slices. In a mixing bowl, mix the flour, olive oil, water, and eggplants.
2. Slowly coat the eggplants. Add eggplants to the air fryer and cook for 12 minutes. Serve with yogurt or tomato sauce.

Nutrition:

- Calories: 103
- Total Fat: 7.3 g
- Carbs: 12.3 g
- Protein: 1.9 g

157. Charred Bell Peppers

Preparation Time: 7 minutes

Cooking Time: 4 minutes

Servings: 3

Ingredients:

- 20 bell peppers, sliced and seeded
- 1 tsp. olive oil
- 1 pinch sea salt
- 1 lemon
- Pepper

Directions:

1. Preheat your air fryer to 390°F. Sprinkle the peppers with oil and salt. Cook the peppers in the air fryer for 4 minutes.
2. Place peppers in a large bowl, and squeeze lemon juice over the top. Season with salt and pepper.

Nutrition:

- Calories: 30
- Total Fat: 0.25 g
- Carbs: 6.91 g
- Protein: 1.28 g

158. Garlic Tomatoes

Preparation Time: 7 minutes

Cooking Time: 15 minutes

Servings: 4

Ingredients:

- 3 tbsp. vinegar
- 1/2 tsp. thyme, dried
- 4 tomatoes
- 1 tbsp. olive oil
- Salt and black pepper to taste
- 1 garlic clove, minced

Directions:

1. Preheat your air fryer to 390°F. Scratch the tomatoes into halves and remove the seeds. Please place them in a big bowl and toss them with oil, salt, pepper, garlic, and thyme.
2. Place them into the air fryer and cook for 15 minutes. Drizzle with vinegar and serve.

Nutrition:

- Calories: 28.9
- Total Fat: 2.4 g
- Carbs: 2.0 g
- Protein: 0.4 g

159. Mushroom Stew

Preparation Time: 7 minutes

Cooking Time: 1 hour 22 minutes

Servings: 3

Ingredients:

- 1 lb. chicken, cubed, boneless, skinless
- 2 tbsp. canola oil
- 1 lb. fresh mushrooms, sliced
- 1 tbsp. thyme, dried
- 1/4 cup water
- 2 tbsp. tomato paste
- 4 garlic cloves, minced
- 1 cup green peppers, sliced
- 3 cups zucchini, diced
- 1 large onion, diced
- 1 tbsp. basil
- 1 tbsp. marjoram
- 1 tbsp. oregano

Directions:

1. Cut the chicken into cubes. Position them in the air fryer basket and pour olive oil over them. Add mushrooms, zucchini, onion, and green pepper. Mix and add garlic, cook for 2 minutes, then add tomato paste, water, and seasonings.
2. Lock the air fryer and cook the stew for 50 minutes. Set the heat to 340°F and cook for an additional 20 minutes.
3. Remove from air fryer and transfer into a large pan. Empty in a bit of water and simmer for 10 minutes.

Nutrition:

- Calories: 53
- Total Fat: 3.3 g
- Carbs: 4.9 g
- Protein: 2.3 g

160.   Cheese & Onion Nuggets

Preparation Time: 7 minutes

Cooking Time: 12 minutes

Servings: 4

Ingredients:

- 7 oz. Edam cheese, grated
- 2 spring onions, diced
- 1 egg, beaten
- 1 tbsp. coconut oil
- 1 tbsp. thyme, dried
- Salt and pepper to taste

Directions:

1. Mix the onion, cheese, coconut oil, salt, pepper, thyme in a bowl. Make 8 small balls and place the cheese in the center.
2. Place in the fridge for about an hour. With a pastry brush, carefully brush the beaten egg over the nuggets. Cook for 12 minutes in the air fryer at 350°F.

Nutrition:

- Calories: 227
- Total Fat: 17.3 g
- Carbs: 4.5 g
- Protein: 14.2 g

161.   Spiced Nuts

Preparation Time: 7 minutes

Cooking Time: 25 minutes

Servings: 3

Ingredients:

- 1 cup almonds
- 1 cup pecan halves
- 1 cup cashews
- 1 egg white, beaten
- 1/2 tsp. cinnamon, ground
- Pinch cayenne pepper
- 1/4 tsp. cloves, ground
- Pinch salt

Directions:

1. Combine the egg white with spices. Preheat your air fryer to 300ºF.
2. Toss the nuts in the spiced mixture. Cook for 25 minutes, stirring several times throughout cooking time.

Nutrition:

- Calories: 88.4
- Total Fat: 7.6 g
- Carbs: 3.9 g
- Protein: 2.5 g

162.   Keto French fries

Preparation Time: 7 minutes

Cooking Time: 20 minutes

Servings: 4

Ingredients:

- 1 large rutabaga, peeled, cut into spears about ¼-inch wide
- Salt and pepper to taste
- 1/2 tsp. paprika
- 2 tbsp. coconut oil

Directions:

1. Preheat your air fryer to 450ºF. Mix the oil, paprika, salt, and pepper.
2. Pour the oil mixture over the rutabaga fries, making sure all pieces are well coated. Cook in the air fryer for 20 minutes or until crispy.

Nutrition:

- Calories: 113
- Total Fat: 7.2 g
- Carbs: 12.5 g
- Protein: 1.9 g

163.   Fried Garlic Green Tomatoes

Preparation Time: 7 minutes

Cooking Time: 12 minutes

Servings: 2

Ingredients:

- 3 green tomatoes, sliced
- 1/2 cup almond flour
- 2 eggs, beaten
- Salt and pepper to taste
- 1 tsp. garlic, minced

Directions:

1. Season the tomatoes with salt, garlic, and pepper. Preheat your air fryer to 400°F. Dip the tomatoes first in flour then in the egg mixture.
2. Spray the tomato rounds with olive oil and place them in the air fryer basket. Cook for 8 minutes, then flip over and cook for additional 4 minutes. Serve with zero-carb mayonnaise.

Nutrition:

- Calories: 123
- Total Fat: 3.9 g
- Carbs: 16 g
- Protein: 8.4 g

164.   Garlic Cauliflower Tots

Preparation Time: 7 minutes

Cooking Time: 20 minutes

Servings: 4

Ingredients:

- 1 crown cauliflower, chopped in a food processor
- 1/2 cup parmesan cheese, grated
- Salt and pepper to taste
- 1/4 cup almond flour
- 2 eggs
- 1 tsp. garlic, minced

Directions:

1. Mix all the ingredients. Shape into tots and spray with olive oil. Preheat your air fryer to 400°F.
2. Cook for 10 minutes on each side.

Nutrition:

- Calories: 18
- Total Fat: 0.6 g
- Carbs: 1.3 g
- Protein: 1.8 g

CHAPTER 16.
DESSERTS AND
SNACKS RECIPES

102.   Apple Crisp

Preparation time: 20 minutes

Cooking time: 30 minutes

Servings: 2

Ingredients:

- 5 cups Granny Smith apples, peeled and sliced
- 3 tbsp. margarine
- 1/2 cup rolled oats
- 1/4 cup + 2 tbsp. Splenda
- 3 tbsp. flour
- 1 tsp. lemon juice
- 3/4 tsp. apple pie spice, divided

Directions:

1. Heat oven to 375°F.
2. In a large bowl, combine apples, 2 tbsp. Splenda, lemon juice, and 1/2 tsp. apple pie spice. Mix to thoroughly coat apples.
3. Place apples in a 2 qt. square baking pan.
4. In a medium bowl, combine oats, flour, 1/4 Splenda, and remaining apple pie spice. With a pastry knife, cut in butter until the mixture resembles coarse crumbs. Sprinkle evenly over apples.
5. Bake 30 to 35 minutes, or until apples are tender and topping is golden brown. Serve warm.

Nutrition:

- Calories: 153
- Carbohydrates: 27 g
- Net carbohydrates: 23 g
- Protein: 1 g
- Fat: 5 g
- Sugar: 18 g
- Fiber: 4 g

103.   Apple Pear and Pecan Dessert Squares

Preparation time: 10 minutes

Cooking time: 25 minutes

Servings: 4

Ingredients:

- 1 Granny Smith apple, sliced, leave the peel on
- 1 Red Delicious apple, sliced, leave the peel on
- 1 ripe pear, sliced, leave the peel on
- 3 eggs
- 1/2 cup plain fat-free yogurt

- 1 tbsp. lemon juice
- 1 tbsp. margarine
- 1 package spice cake mix
- 1 1/4 cup water, divided
- 1/2 cup pecan pieces
- 1 tbsp. Splenda
- 1 tsp. cinnamon
- 1/2 tsp. vanilla
- 1/4 tsp. nutmeg
- Non-stick cooking spray

Directions:

1. Heat oven to 350°F. Spray jelly-roll pan with non-stick cooking spray.
2. In a large bowl, beat cake mix, 1 cup water, eggs, and yogurt until smooth. Pour into a prepared pan and bake for 20 minutes or it passes the toothpick test. Cool completely.
3. In a large non-stick skillet, over med-high heat, toast the pecans, stirring, about 2 minutes or until lightly browned. Remove to a plate.
4. Add the remaining 1/4 cup water, sliced fruits, juice, and spices to the skillet. Bring to a boil. Reduce heat to medium and cook 3 minutes or until fruit is tender-crisp.
5. Remove from heat and stir in Splenda, margarine, vanilla, and pecans. Spoon evenly over cooled cake.

Nutrition:

- Calories: 130
- Carbohydrates: 20 g
- Net carbohydrates: 19 g
- Protein: 2 g
- Fat: 5 g
- Sugar: 10 g
- Fiber: 1 g

104.   Apricot Soufflé

Preparation time: 5 minutes

Cooking time: 30 minutes

Servings: 4

Ingredients:

- 4 egg whites
- 3 egg yolks, beaten
- 3 tbsp. margarine
- 3/4 cup sugar-free apricot fruit spread
- 1/3 cup dried apricots, diced fine
- 1/4 cup warm water
- 2 tbsp. flour
- 1/4 tsp. cream of tartar
- 1/8 tsp. salt

Directions:

1. Heat oven to 325°F.

2. In a medium saucepan, over medium heat, melt margarine. Stir in flour and cook, stirring, until bubbly.

3. Stir together the fruit spread and water in a small bowl and add it to the saucepan with the apricots. Cook, stirring, 3 minutes or until mixture thickens.

4. Remove from heat and whisk in egg yolks. Let cool to room temperature, stirring occasionally.

5. In a medium bowl, beat egg whites, salt, and cream of tartar at high speed until stiff peaks form. Gently fold into cooled apricot mixture.

6. Spoon into a 1 1/2 qt. soufflé dish. Bake 30 minutes, or until puffed and golden brown.

Nutrition:

- Calories: 116
- Carbohydrates: 7 g
- Protein: 4 g
- Fat: 8 g
- Sugar: 1 g
- Fiber: 0 g

105. Autumn Skillet Cake

Preparation time: 10 minutes

Cooking time: 30 minutes

Servings: 4

Ingredients:

- 3 eggs, room temperature
- 1 cup fresh cranberries
- 4 oz. cream cheese, soft
- 3 tbsp. fat-free sour cream
- 2 tbsp. butter, melted
- 2 cups almond flour, sifted
- 3/4 cup Splenda
- 3/4 cup pumpkin puree
- 1 1/2 tbsp. baking powder
- 2 tsp. cinnamon
- 1 tsp. pumpkin spice
- 1 tsp. ginger
- 1/4 tsp. nutmeg
- 1/4 tsp. salt
- Non-stick cooking spray

Directions:

1. Heat oven to 350°F. Spray a 9-inch cast-iron skillet or cake pan with cooking spray.

2. In a large bowl, beat Splenda, butter, and cream cheese until thoroughly combined. Add eggs, one at a time, beating after each.

3. Add pumpkin and spices and combine. Add the dry ingredients and mix well. Stir in the sour cream. Pour into a prepared pan.

4. Sprinkle cranberries over the batter and with the back of a spoon, push them

halfway into the batter. Bake 30 minutes or the cake passes the toothpick test. Cool completely before serving.

Nutrition:

- Calories: 280
- Carbohydrates: 23 g
- Net carbohydrates: 20 g
- Protein: 7 g
- Fat: 17 g
- Sugar: 16 g
- Fiber: 3 g

106. Baked Maple Custard

Preparation time: 5 minutes

Cooking time: 1 hour 15 minutes

Servings: 2

Ingredients:

- 2 1/2 cup half-and-half
- 1/2 cup egg substitute
- 3 cup boiling water
- 1/4 cup Splenda
- 2 tbsp. sugar-free maple syrup
- 2 tsp. vanilla
- A dash of nutmeg
- Non-stick cooking spray

Directions:

1. Heat oven to 325°F. Lightly spray 6 custard cups or ramekins with cooking spray.

2. In a large bowl, whisk together half-n-half, egg substitute, Splenda, vanilla, and nutmeg. Pour evenly into prepared custard cups. Place cups in a 13x9-inch baking dish.

3. Pour boiling water around, being careful not to splash it into, the cups. Bake 1 hour 15 minutes, centers will not be completely set.

4. Remove cups from the pan and cool completely. Cover and chill overnight.

5. Just before serving, drizzle with the maple syrup.

Nutrition:

- Calories: 190
- Carbohydrates: 15 g
- Protein: 5 g
- Fat: 12 g
- Sugar: 8 g
- Fiber: 0 g

107. Blackberry Crostata

Preparation time: 10 minutes

Cooking time: 20 minutes

Servings: 3

Ingredients:

- 1 9-inch pie crust, unbaked
- 2 cup fresh blackberries
- Juice and zest of 1 lemon
- 2 tbsp. butter, soft
- 3 tbsp. Splenda, divided
- 2 tbsp. cornstarch

Directions:

1. Heat oven to 425°F. Line a large baking sheet with parchment paper and unroll pie crust in the pan.
2. In a medium bowl, combine blackberries, 2 tbsp. Splenda, lemon juice and zest, and cornstarch. Spoon onto crust leaving a 2-inch edge. Fold and crimp the edges.
3. Dot the berries with 1 tbsp. butter. Brush the crust edge with remaining butter and sprinkle crust and fruit with remaining Splenda.
4. Bake 20 to 22 minutes or until golden brown. Cool before cutting and serving.

Nutrition:

- Calories: 206
- Carbohydrates: 24 g
- Net carbohydrates: 21 g
- Protein: 2 g
- Fat: 11 g

- Sugar: 9 g
- Fiber: 3 g

108.   Blackberry Soufflés

Preparation time: 15 minutes

Cooking time: 30 minutes

Servings: 4

Ingredients:

- 12 oz. blackberries
- 4 egg whites
- 1/3 cup Splenda
- 1 tbsp. water
- 1 tbsp. Swerve powdered sugar
- Non-stick cooking spray

Directions:

1. Heat oven to 375°F. Spray 4 1 cup ramekins with cooking spray.
2. In a small saucepan, over med-high heat, combine blackberries and 1 tbsp. water, bring to a boil. Reduce heat and simmer until berries are soft. Add Splenda and stir over medium heat until Splenda dissolves, without boiling.
3. Bring back to boiling, reduce heat and simmer for 5 minutes. Remove from heat and cool for 5 minutes.

4. Place a fine-meshed sieve over a small bowl and push the berry mixture through it using the back of a spoon. Discard the seeds. Cover and chill for 15 minutes.

5. In a large bowl, beat egg whites until soft peaks form. Gently fold in berry mixture. Spoon evenly into prepared ramekins and place them on a baking sheet.

6. Bake 12 minutes, or until puffed and light brown. Dust with powdered Swerve and serve immediately.

Nutrition:

- Calories: 141
- Carbohydrates: 26 g
- Net carbohydrates: 21 g
- Protein: 5 g
- Fat: 0 g
- Sugar: 20 g
- Fiber: 5 g

109.   Blueberry Lemon "Cup" Cakes

Preparation time: 5 minutes

Cooking time: 10 minutes

Servings: 2

Ingredients:

- 4 eggs
- 1/2 cup coconut milk
- 1/2 cup blueberries
- 2 tbsp. lemon zest
- 1/2 cup + 1 tsp. coconut flour
- 1/4 cup Splenda
- 1/4 cup coconut oil, melted
- 1 tsp. baking soda
- 1/2 tsp. lemon extract
- 1/4 tsp. Stevia extract
- A pinch of salt

Directions:

1. In a small bowl, toss blueberries in 1 tsp. flour.

2. In a large bowl, stir together the remaining flour, Splenda, baking soda, salt, and zest.

3. Add the remaining ingredients and mix well. Fold in the blueberries.

4. Divide batter evenly into 5 coffee cups. Microwave, one at a time, for 90 seconds, or until they pass the toothpick test.

Nutrition:

- Calories: 263
- Carbohydrates: 14 g
- Net carbohydrates: 12 g
- Protein: 5 g
- Fat: 20 g
- Sugar: 12 g
- Fiber: 2 g

110.   Blueberry No Bake Cheesecake

Preparation time: 5 minutes

Cooking time: 3 Hours

Servings: 3

Ingredients:

- 16 oz. fat-free cream cheese softened
- 1 cup sugar-free frozen whipped topping, thawed
- 3/4 cup blueberries
- 1 tbsp. margarine, melted
- 8 Zwieback toasts
- 1 cup boiling water
- 1/3 cup Splenda
- 1 envelope unflavored gelatin
- 1 tsp. vanilla

Directions:

1. Place the toasts and margarine in a food processor. Pulse until mixture resembles coarse crumbs. Press on the bottom of a 9-inch springform pan.
2. Place gelatin in a medium bowl and add boiling water. Stir until gelatin dissolved completely.
3. In a large bowl, beat cream cheese, Splenda, and vanilla on medium speed until well blended. Beat in whipped topping. Add gelatin, in a steady stream, while beating at low speed. Increase speed to medium and beat 4 minutes or until smooth and creamy.
4. Gently fold in blueberries and spread over crust. Cover and chill for 3 hours or until set.

Nutrition:

- Calories: 316
- Carbohydrates: 20 g
- Protein: 6 g
- Fat: 23 g
- Sugar: 10 g
- Fiber: 0 g

111.   Broiled Stone Fruit

Preparation time: 5 minutes

Cooking time: 5 minutes

Servings: 2

Ingredients:

- 1 peach
- 1 nectarine
- 2 tbsp. sugar-free whipped topping
- 1 tbsp. Splenda brown sugar
- Non-stick cooking spray

Directions:

1. Heat oven to broil. Line a shallow baking dish with foil and spray with cooking spray.
2. Cut the peach and nectarine in half and remove pits. Place cut side down in prepared dish. Broil 3 minutes.
3. Turn the fruit over and sprinkle with Splenda brown sugar. Broil another 2 to 3 minutes.
4. Transfer 1 of each fruit to a dessert bowl and top with 1 tbsp. whipped topping.

Nutrition:

- Calories: 101
- Carbohydrates: 22 g
- Net carbohydrates: 20 g
- Protein: 1 g
- Fat: 1 g
- Sugar: 19 g
- Fiber: 2 g

112.   Café Mocha Torte

Preparation time: 15 minutes

Cooking time: 25 minutes

Servings: 4

Ingredients:

- 8 eggs
- 1 cup margarine, cut into cubes
- 1 lb. bittersweet chocolate, chopped
- 1/4 cup brewed coffee, room temperature
- Non-stick cooking spray
- 2 cups water

Directions:

1. Heat oven to 325°F. Spray an 8-inch springform pan with cooking spray. Line bottom of sides with parchment paper and spray again. Wrap the outside with a double layer of foil and place in a 9x13-inch baking dish. Put a small saucepan of water on to boil.
2. In a large bowl, beat the eggs on med speed until doubled in volume, about 5 minutes.
3. Place the chocolate, margarine, and coffee into a microwave-safe bowl and microwave on high, until chocolate is melted, and mixture is smooth, stirring every 30 seconds.
4. Fold 1/3 of the eggs into a chocolate mixture until almost combined. Add the remaining eggs, 1/3 at a time, and fold until combined.
5. Pour into a prepared pan. Pour boiling water around the springform pan until it reaches halfway up the sides. Bake 22 to 25 minutes, or until the cake has risen slightly and edges are just beginning to set.

6. Remove from water bath and let cool completely. Cover with plastic wrap and chill 6 hours or overnight. About 30 minutes before serving, run a knife around the edges and remove the side of the pan. Slice and serve.

Nutrition:

- Calories: 260
- Carbohydrates: 12 g
- Net carbohydrates: 11 g
- Protein: 5 g
- Fat: 21 g
- Sugar: 11 g
- Fiber: 1 g

113. Cappuccino Mousse

Preparation time: 5 minutes

Cooking time: 1 Hour

Servings: 3

Ingredients:

- 2 cups low fat cream cheese, soft
- 1 cup half-n-half
- 1/2 cup almond milk, unsweetened
- 1/4 cup strong brewed coffee, cooled completely
- 1–2 tsp. coffee extract
- 1 tsp. vanilla liquid sweetener
- Whole coffee beans for garnish

Directions:

1. In a large bowl, beat cream cheese and coffee on high speed until smooth. Add milk, 1 tsp. coffee extract, and liquid sweetener. Beat until smooth and thoroughly combined.
2. Pour in half-n-half and continue beating until the mixture resembles the texture of mousse.
3. Spoon into dessert glasses or ramekins, cover, and chill at least 1 hour before serving. Garnish with a coffee bean and serve.

Nutrition:

- Calories: 98
- Carbohydrates: 5 g
- Protein: 9 g
- Fat: 5 g
- Sugar: 0 g
- Fiber: 0 g

114. Caramel Pecan Pie

Preparation time: 5 minutes

Cooking time: 35 minutes

Servings: 2

Ingredients:

- 1 cup pecans, chopped
- 3/4 cup almond milk, unsweetened
- 1/3 cup margarine, melted
- 2 cup almond flour
- 1/2 cup + 2 tbsp. Splenda for baking
- 1 tsp. vanilla
- 1 tsp. Arrowroot powder
- 3/4 tsp. sea salt
- 1/2 tsp. vanilla
- 1/2 tsp. maple syrup, sugar-free
- Non-stick cooking spray

Directions:

1. Heat oven to 350°F. Spray a 9-inch pie pan with cooking spray.

2. In a medium bowl, combine flour, melted margarine, 2 tbsp. Splenda, and vanilla. Mix to thoroughly combine ingredients. Press on the bottom and sides of a prepared pie pan. Bake 12–15 minutes, or until edges start to brown. Set aside.

3. In a small saucepan, combine milk, remaining Splenda, arrowroot, salt, 1/2 tsp. vanilla, and syrup. Cook over medium heat until it starts to boil, stirring constantly. Keep cooking until it turns a gold color and starts to thicken about 2 to 3 minutes. Remove from heat and let cool. Stir in 1/2 of the pecans.

4. Pour the filling in the crust and top with the remaining pecans. Bake about 15 minutes, or until the filling starts to bubble. Cool completely before serving.

Nutrition:

- Calories: 375
- Carbohydrates: 20 g
- Net carbohydrates: 15 g
- Protein: 7 g
- Fat: 30 g
- Sugar: 14 g
- Fiber: 5 g

115.   Carrot Cupcakes

Preparation time: 10 minutes

Cooking time: 35 minutes

Servings: 2

Ingredients:

- 2 cup carrots, grated
- 1 cup low fat cream cheese, soft
- 2 eggs
- 1–2 tsp. skim milk
- 1/2 cup coconut oil, melted
- 1/4 cup coconut flour
- 1/4 cup Splenda
- 1/4 cup honey
- 2 tsp. vanilla, divided

- 1 tsp. baking powder
- 1 tsp. cinnamon
- Non-stick cooking spray

Directions:

1. Heat oven to 350°F. Lightly spray a muffin pan with cooking spray, or use paper liners.
2. In a large bowl, stir together the flour, baking powder, and cinnamon.
3. Add the carrots, eggs, oil, Splenda, and vanilla to a food processor. Process until ingredients are combined but carrots still have some large chunks remaining. Add to dry ingredients and stir to combine.
4. Pour evenly into prepared pan, filling cups 2/3 full. Bake 30 to 35 minutes, or until cupcakes pass the toothpick test. Remove from oven and let cool.
5. In a medium bowl, beat cream cheese, honey, and vanilla on high speed until smooth. Add milk, one tsp. at a time, beating after each addition, until frosting is creamy enough to spread easily.
6. Once cupcakes have cooled, spread each one with about 2 tbsp. frosting. Chill until ready to serve.

Nutrition:

- Calories: 160
- Carbohydrates: 13 g
- Net carbohydrates: 12 g
- Protein: 4 g
- Fat: 10 g
- Sugar: 11 g
- Fiber: 1 g

116. Chocolate Cherry Cake Roll

Preparation time: 10 minutes

Cooking time: 15 minutes

Servings: 4

Ingredients:

- 10 maraschino cherries, drained and patted dry
- 4 eggs, room temperature
- 1 cup sugar-free Cool Whip, thawed
- 2/3 cup maraschino cherries, chop, drain and pat dry
- 1/2 cup cream cheese, soft
- 1/3 cup flour
- 1/2 cup Splenda for baking
- 1/4 cup unsweetened cocoa powder
- 1 tbsp. sugar-free hot fudge ice cream topping
- 1/4 tsp. baking soda
- 1/4 tsp. salt
- Unsweetened cocoa powder
- Non-stick cooking spray

Directions:

1. Heat oven to 375°F. Spray a large sheet baking pan with cooking spray. Line bottom with parchment paper, spray and flour the paper.

2. In a small bowl, stir together flour, 1/4 cup cocoa, baking soda, and salt.

3. In a large bowl, beat eggs on high speed for 5 minutes,

4. Gradually add sweetener and continue beating until the mixture is thick and lemon colored.

5. Fold in dry ingredients. Spread evenly into the prepared pan. Bake 15 minutes or top springs back when touched lightly.

6. Place a clean towel on a cutting board and sprinkle with cocoa powder. Turn the cake onto the towel and carefully remove parchment paper.

7. Starting at a short end, roll up the towel. Cool on a wire rack for 1 hour.

8. Prepare the filling: In a small bowl, beat cream cheese until smooth. Add 1/2 cup whipped topping, beat on low until combined. Fold in another 1/2 cup whipped topping. Fold in the chopped cherries.

9. Unroll the cake and remove the towel. Spread the filling to within 1-inch of the edges. Reroll cake and trim the ends. Cover and chill for at least 2 hours or overnight.

10. To serve, warm up the fudge topping and drizzle over cake, garnish with whole cherries, then slice and serve.

Nutrition:

- Calories: 163
- Carbohydrates: 25 g
- Protein: 5 g
- Fat: 3 g
- Sugar: 12 g
- Fiber: 0 g

117.   Chocolate Orange Bread Pudding

Preparation time: 10 minutes

Cooking time: 35 minutes

Servings: 4

Ingredients:

- 4 cups French baguette cubes
- 1 1/2 cups skim milk
- 3 eggs, lightly beaten
- 1–2 tsp. orange zest, grated
- 1/4 cup Splenda
- 1/4 cup sugar-free chocolate ice cream topping
- 3 tbsp. unsweetened cocoa powder
- 1 tsp. vanilla
- 3/4 tsp. cinnamon

Directions:

1. Heat oven to 350°F.
2. In a medium bowl, stir together Splenda and cocoa. Stir in milk, eggs, zest, vanilla, and cinnamon until well blended.
3. Place bread cubes in an 8-inch square baking dish. Pour milk mixture evenly over the top.
4. Bake 35 minutes or until a knife inserted in the center comes out clean. Cool 5 to 10 minutes.
5. Spoon into dessert dishes and drizzle lightly with ice cream topping.

Nutrition:

- Calories: 139
- Carbohydrates: 23 g
- Net carbohydrates: 22 g
- Protein: 6 g
- Fat: 2 g
- Sugar: 9 g
- Fiber: 1 g

118. Chocolate Torte

Preparation time: 15 minutes

Cooking time: 35 minutes

Servings: 4

Ingredients:

- 5 eggs, separated, room temperature
- 3/4 cup margarine, sliced
- 1 package. semisweet chocolate chips
- 1/2 cup Splenda
- 1/4 tsp. cream of tartar
- Non-stick cooking spray
- 1/4 of egg whites

Directions:

1. Heat oven to 350°F. Spray a 6–7-inch springform pan with cooking spray.
2. In a microwave-safe bowl, melt chocolate chips and margarine, in 30-second intervals.
3. In a large bowl, beat egg yolks till thick and lemon-colored. Beat in chocolate.
4. In a separate large bowl, with clean beaters, beat egg whites and cream of tartar till foamy. Beat in Splenda, 1 tbsp. at a time, till sugar is dissolved, continue beating till stiff glossy peaks form.
5. Fold 1/4 of egg whites into the chocolate mixture, then fold in the rest. Transfer to prepared pan. Bake 30 to 35 minutes or the center is set. Let cool completely before removing the side of the pan and serving.

Nutrition:

- Calories: 181
- Carbohydrates: 10 g
- Protein: 3 g
- Fat: 14 g
- Sugar: 10 g
- Fiber: 0 g

119.   Cinnamon Bread Pudding

Preparation time: 10 minutes

Cooking time: 45 minutes

Servings: 2

Ingredients:

- 4 cups day-old French or Italian bread, cut into 3/4-inch cubes
- 2 cups skim milk
- 2 egg whites
- 1 egg
- 4 tbsp. margarine, sliced
- 5 tsp. Splenda
- 1 1/2 tsp. cinnamon
- 1/4 tsp. salt
- 1/8 tsp. ground cloves
- 1-inch of hot water

Directions:

1. Heat oven to 350°F.
2. In a medium saucepan, heat milk and margarine to simmering. Remove from heat and stir till margarine is completely melted. Let cool for 10 minutes.
3. In a large bowl, beat egg and egg whites until foamy. Add Splenda, spices, and salt. Beat until combined, then add in cooled milk and bread.
4. Transfer mixture to a 1 1/2 qt. baking dish. Place on rack of roasting pan and add 1-inch of hot water to the roaster.
5. Bake until pudding is set and a knife inserted in the center comes out clean, about 40 to 45 minutes.

Nutrition:

- Calories: 362
- Carbohydrates: 25 g
- Net carbohydrates: 23 g
- Protein: 14 g
- Fat: 10 g
- Sugar: 10 g
- Fiber: 2 g

120.   Coconut Cream Pie

Preparation time: 5 minutes

Cooking time: 10 minutes

Servings: 2

Ingredients:

- 2 cups raw coconut, grated and divided
- 2 cans coconut milk, full fat, and refrigerated for 24 hours
- 1/2 cup raw coconut, grated and toasted
- 2 tbsp. margarine, melted
- 1 cup Splenda
- 1/2 cup macadamia nuts
- 1/4 cup almond flour
- 1 cup water

Directions:

1. Heat oven to 350°F.
2. Add the nuts to a food processor and pulse until finely ground. Add flour, 1/2 cup Splenda, and 1 cup grated coconut. Pulse until ingredients are finely ground and resemble cracker crumbs.
3. Add the margarine and pulse until the mixture starts to stick together. Press on the bottom and sides of a 9-inch pie pan. Bake 10 minutes or until golden brown. Cool
4. Turn the canned coconut upside down and open. Pour off the water and scoop the cream into a large bowl. Add remaining 1/2 cup Splenda and beat on high until stiff peaks form.

5. Fold in the remaining 1 cup coconut and pour into crust. Cover and chill for at least 2 hours. Sprinkle with toasted coconut, slice, and serve.

Nutrition:

- Calories: 329
- Carbohydrates: 15 g
- Net carbohydrates: 4 g
- Protein: 4 g
- Fat: 23 g
- Sugar: 4 g
- Fiber: 11 g

121.   Coconut Milk Shakes

Preparation time: 5 minutes

Cooking time: 5 minutes

Servings: 2

Ingredients:

- 1 1/2 cup vanilla ice cream
- 1/2 cup coconut milk, unsweetened
- 2 1/2 tbsp. coconut flakes
- 1 tsp. unsweetened cocoa

Directions:

1. Heat oven to 350°F.

2. Place coconut on a baking sheet and bake, 2 to 3 minutes, stirring often, until coconut is toasted.

3. Place ice cream, milk, 2 tbsp. coconut, and cocoa in a blender and process until smooth.

4. Pour into glasses and garnish with remaining toasted coconut. Serve immediately.

Nutrition:

- Calories: 323
- Carbohydrates: 23 g
- Net carbohydrates: 19 g
- Protein: 3 g
- Fat: 24 g
- Sugar: 18 g
- Fiber: 4 g

122. Cheesy Pita Crisps

Preparation time: 5 minutes

Cooking time: 15 minutes

Servings: 4

Ingredients:

- 1/2 cup mozzarella cheese
- 1/4 cup margarine, melted
- 4 whole-wheat pita pocket halves
- 3 tbsp. reduced-fat parmesan
- 1/2 tsp. garlic powder
- 1/2 tsp. onion powder
- 1/4 tsp. salt
- 1/4 tsp. pepper
- Non-stick cooking spray

Directions:

1. Heat oven to 400°F. Spray a baking sheet with cooking spray.

2. Cut each pita pocket in half. Cut each half into 2 triangles. Place, rough side up, on prepared pan.

3. In a small bowl, whisk together margarine, parmesan, and seasonings. Spread each triangle with a margarine mixture. Sprinkle mozzarella over top.

4. Bake 12 to 15 minutes or until golden brown.

Nutrition:

- Calories: 131
- Carbohydrates: 14 g
- Net carbohydrates: 12 g
- Protein: 4 g
- Fat: 7 g
- Sugar: 1 g
- Fiber: 2 g

123. Cheesy Taco Chips

Preparation time: 15 minutes

Cooking time: 40 minutes

Servings: 2

Ingredients:

- 1 cup Mexican blend cheese, grated
- 2 large egg whites
- 1 1/2 cup crushed pork rinds
- 1 tbsp. taco seasoning
- 1/4 tsp. salt

Directions:

1. Heat oven to 300°F. Line a large baking sheet with parchment paper.
2. In a large bowl, whisk egg whites and salt until frothy. Stir in pork rinds, cheese, and seasoning and stir until thoroughly combined.
3. Turn out onto the prepared pan. Place another sheet of parchment paper on top and roll out very thin, about 12x12-inches. Remove top sheet of parchment paper, and using a pizza cutter, score dough in 2-inch squares, then score each square in half diagonally.
4. Bake 20 minutes until they start to brown. Turn off the oven and let them sit inside the oven until they are firm to the touch, about 10 to 20 minutes.
5. Remove from oven and cool completely before breaking apart. Eat them as is or with your favorite dip.

Nutrition:

- Calories: 260
- Carbohydrates: 1 g
- Protein: 25 g
- Fat: 17 g
- Sugar: 0 g
- Fiber: 0 g

124. Chewy Granola Bars

Preparation time: 10 minutes

Cooking time: 35 minutes

Servings: 3

Ingredients:

- 1 egg, beaten
- 2/3 cup margarine, melted
- 3 1/2 cup quick oats
- 1 cup almonds, chopped
- 1/2 cup honey
- 1/2 cup sunflower kernels
- 1/2 cup coconut, unsweetened
- 1/2 cup dried apples

- 1/2 cup dried cranberries
- 1/2 cup Splenda brown sugar
- 1 tsp. vanilla
- 1/2 tsp. cinnamon
- Non-stick cooking spray

Directions:

1. Heat oven to 350°F. Spray a large baking sheet with cooking spray.
2. Spread oats and almonds on a prepared pan. Bake 12 to 15 minutes until toasted, stirring every few minutes.
3. In a large bowl, combine egg, margarine, honey, and vanilla. Stir in remaining ingredients.
4. Stir in oat mixture. Press into baking sheet and bake 13 to 18 minutes, or until edges are light brown.
5. Cool on a wire rack. Cut into bars and store in an airtight container.

Nutrition:

- Calories: 119
- Carbohydrates: 13 g
- Net carbohydrates: 12 g
- Protein: 2 g
- Fat: 6 g
- Sugar: 7 g
- Fiber: 1 g

125. Chili Lime Tortilla Chips

Preparation time: 5 minutes

Cooking time: 15 minutes

Servings: 4

Ingredients:

- 12–6-inch corn tortillas, cut into 8 triangles
- 3 tbsp. lime juice
- 1 tsp. cumin
- 1 tsp. chili powder

Directions:

1. Heat oven to 350°F.
2. Place tortilla triangles in a single layer on a large baking sheet.
3. In a small bowl, stir together spices.
4. Sprinkle half the lime juice over tortillas, followed by 1/2 the spice mixture. Bake 7 minutes.
5. Remove from oven and turn tortillas over. Sprinkle with remaining lime juice and spices. Bake another 8 minutes or until crisp, but not brown. Serve with your favorite salsa; the serving size is 10 chips.

Nutrition:

- Calories: 65
- Carbohydrates: 14 g

- Net carbohydrates: 12 g
- Protein: 2 g
- Fat: 1 g
- Sugar: 0 g
- Fiber: 2 g

126. Chocolate Chip Blondies

Preparation time: 5 minutes

Cooking time: 20 minutes

Servings: 4

Ingredients:

- 1 egg
- 1/2 cup semi-sweet chocolate chips
- 1/3 cup flour
- 1/3 cup whole wheat flour
- 1/4 cup Splenda brown sugar
- 1/4 cup sunflower oil
- 2 tbsp. honey
- 1 tsp. vanilla
- 1/2 tsp. baking powder
- 1/4 tsp. salt
- Non-stick cooking spray

Directions:

1. Heat oven to 350°F. Spray an 8-inch square baking dish with cooking spray.
2. In a small bowl, combine dry ingredients.
3. In a large bowl, whisk together egg, oil, honey, and vanilla. Stir in dry ingredients just until combined. Stir in chocolate chips.
4. Spread batter in prepared dish. Bake 20 to 22 minutes or until they pass the toothpick test. Cool on a wire rack, then cut into bars.

Nutrition:

- Calories: 136
- Carbohydrates: 18 g
- Net carbohydrates: 16 g
- Protein: 2 g
- Fat: 6 g
- Sugar: 9 g
- Fiber: 2 g

127. Cinnamon Apple Chips

Preparation time: 5 minutes

Cooking time: 10 minutes

Servings: 2

Ingredients:

- 1 medium apple, sliced thin
- 1/4 tsp. cinnamon
- 1/4 tsp. nutmeg
- Non-stick cooking spray

Directions:

1. Heat oven to 375°F. Spray a baking sheet with cooking spray.
2. Place apples in a mixing bowl and add spices. Toss to coat.
3. Arrange apples, in a single layer, on the prepared pan. Bake 4 minutes, turn apples over and bake 4 minutes more.
4. Serve immediately or store in an airtight container.

Nutrition:

- Calories: 58
- Carbohydrates: 15 g
- Protein: 0 g
- Fat: 0 g
- Sugar: 11 g
- Fiber: 3 g

128.   Coffee-Steamed Carrots

Preparation time: 10 minutes

Cooking time: 3 minutes

Servings: 4

Ingredients:

- 1 cup brewed coffee
- 1 tsp. light brown sugar
- 1/2 tsp. kosher salt
- Freshly ground black pepper
- 1 lb. baby carrots
- Chopped fresh parsley
- 1 tsp. grated lemon zest

Directions:

1. Pour the coffee into the electric pressure cooker. Stir in the brown sugar, salt, and pepper. Add the carrots.
2. Close the pressure cooker. Set to sealing.
3. Cook on high pressure for minutes.
4. Once complete, click cancel and quickly release the pressure.
5. Once the pin drops, open and remove the lid.
6. Using a slotted spoon, portion carrots to a serving bowl. Topped with the parsley and lemon zest, and serve.

Nutrition:

- Calories: 51
- Carbohydrates: 12 g
- Fiber: 4 g

129.   Rosemary Potatoes

Preparation time: 5 minutes

Cooking time: 25 minutes

Servings: 2

Ingredients:

- 1 lb. red potatoes
- 1 cup vegetable stock
- 2 tbsp. olive oil
- 2 tbsp. rosemary sprigs

Directions:

1. Situate potatoes in the steamer basket and add the stock into the Instant Pot.
2. Steam the potatoes in your Instant Pot for 15 minutes.
3. Depressurize and pour away the remaining stock.
4. Set to sauté and add the oil, rosemary, and potatoes.
5. Cook until brown.

Nutrition:

- Calories: 195
- Fat: 1 g
- Carbohydrates: 31 g

130. Fantastic Butternut Squash and Vegetables

Preparation time: 15 minutes

Cooking time: 4 hours

Servings: 2

Ingredients:

- 1 1/2 cups corn kernels
- 2 lb. butternut squash
- 1 medium-sized green bell pepper
- 14 1/2 oz. diced tomatoes
- 1/2 cup chopped white onion
- 1/2 tsp. minced garlic
- 1/2 tsp. salt
- 1/4 tsp. ground black pepper
- 1 tbsp. and 2 tsp. tomato paste
- 1/2 cup vegetable broth

Directions:

1. Peel, centralize the butternut squash and dice, and place it into a 6 qt. slow cooker. Create a hole on the green bell pepper, then cut it into 1/2-inch pieces and add it to the slow cooker. Add the remaining ingredients into the slow cooker except for tomato paste, stir properly and cover it with the lid.
2. Turn on the slow cooker and cook on a low heat setting for 6 hours. When 6 hours of the cooking time is done, remove 1/2 cup of the cooking liquid from the slow cooker. Then pour the tomato mixture into this cooking liquid, stir properly and place it in the slow cooker.
3. Stir properly and continue cooking for 30 minutes or until the mixture becomes slightly thick. Serve right away.

Nutrition:

- Calories: 134
- Carbohydrates: 23 g
- Protein: 6 g

131.   Fabulous Glazed Carrots

Preparation time: 20 minutes

Cooking time: 2 hours

Servings: 4

Ingredients:

- 1 lb. carrots
- 2 tsp. chopped cilantro
- 1/4 tsp. salt
- 1/4 cup brown sugar
- 1/4 tsp. ground cinnamon
- 1/8 tsp. ground nutmeg
- 1 tbsp. cornstarch
- 1 tbsp. olive oil
- 2 tbsp. water
- 1 large orange, juiced and zested

Directions:

1. Peel the carrots, rinse, cut them into 1/4-inch-thick rounds and place them in a 6 qt. slow cooker. Add the salt, sugar, cinnamon, nutmeg, olive oil, orange zest, juice, and stir properly.

2. Cover, cook in the slow cooker on high heat setting for 2 hours. Stir properly the cornstarch and water until it blends well. Thereafter, add this mixture to the slow cooker.

3. Continue cooking for 10 minutes or until the sauce in the slow cooker gets slightly thick. Sprinkle the cilantro over carrots and serve.

Nutrition:

- Calories: 160
- Carbohydrates:40 g
- Protein: 1 g

195.   Sweet Potato Fries

Preparation Time: 5 minutes

Cooking Time: 8 minutes

Servings: 4

Ingredients:

- 2 medium sweet potatoes, peeled
- 1 tbsp. arrowroot starch
- 2 tbsp. cinnamon
- 1/4 cup coconut sugar
- 2 tsp. melted butter, unsalted
- 1/2 tbsp. olive oil
- Confectioners swerve as needed

Directions:

1. Switch on the air fryer, insert fryer basket, grease it with olive oil, then shut with its lid, set the fryer to 370°F, and preheat for 5 minutes.

2. Meanwhile, cut peeled sweet potatoes into ½-inch thick slices, place them in a bowl, add oil and starch and toss until well coated.

3. Open the fryer, add sweet potatoes to it, close with its lid, and cook for 8 minutes until nicely golden, shaking halfway through the frying.

4. When the air fryer beeps, open its lid, transfer sweet potato fries in a bowl, add butter, sprinkle with sugar and cinnamon and toss until well mixed.

5. Sprinkle confectioners swerve on the fries and serve.

Nutrition:

- Calories: 130
- Carbs: 27 g
- Fat: 2.3 g
- Protein: 1.2 g
- Fiber: 3 g

196.   Cheese Sticks

Preparation Time: 5−7 minutes

Cooking Time: 5 minutes

Servings: 2

Ingredients:

- 10 pcs. spring roll wrappers, separated, quartered
- 1/4 lb. sharp cheddar cheese, reduced fat, sliced into 2" x ½" matchsticks
- Oil for spraying

Directions:

1. Preheat the air fryer to 400°F.

2. Place cheese matchstick at the widest end of quartered spring roll wrapper. Moisten edges and tip of the wrapper with water. Fold spring roll wrapper over cheese, and tuck in both ends. Roll spring rolls tightly up to the tip. Place this into a freezer-safe container lined with saran wrap. Repeat the step for all cheese and spring roll wrappers.

3. Freeze for 1 hour before frying.

4. Spray a small amount of oil all over cheese matchsticks. Place a generous handful inside the air fryer basket. Fry for 3 to 5 minutes, or only until wrappers turn golden brown. Shake contents of the basket once midway through.

5. Remove from the basket. Set on plates. Repeat the step for the remaining breaded cheese sticks. Serve.

Nutrition:

- Calories: 229
- Carbs: 16 g
- Fat: 10 g
- Protein: 15 g
- Fiber: 1.8 g

197.   Zucchini Crisps

Preparation Time: 30 minutes

Cooking Time: 30 minutes

Servings: 2

Ingredients:

- 2 zucchini, sliced into a 1/8-inch thick disk
- Pinch sea salt
- White pepper to taste
- 1 tbsp. of olive oil for drizzling

Directions:

1. Preheat the air fryer to 330°F.
2. Put zucchini in a bowl with salt. Let it sit in a colander to drain for 30 minutes.
3. Layer zucchini in a baking dish. Drizzle in oil. Season with pepper. Place baking dish in the air fryer basket. Cook for 30 minutes.
4. Adjust seasoning. Serve.

Nutrition:

- Calories: 15.2
- Carbs: 3.6 g

- Fat: 0.1 g
- Protein: 0.6 g
- Fiber: 1.3 g

198.   Tortillas in Green Mango Salsa

Preparation Time: 30 minutes

Cooking Time: 10 minutes

Servings: 4

Ingredients:

Tortillas:

- 4 pcs. corn tortillas
- 1 tbsp. olive oil
- 1/16 tsp. sea salt

Green mango salsa:

- 1 green/unripe mango, minced
- 1 red/ripe Roma tomato, preferably minced
- 1 shallot, peeled, minced
- 1 fresh jalapeno pepper, minced
- 1/4 red bell pepper, minced
- 4 tbsp. fresh cilantro, minced
- 1/4 cup lime juice, freshly squeezed
- 1/16 tsp. salt

Directions:

1. Preheat the air fryer to 400°F.

2. Mix lime juice and salt in a bowl. Stir until solids dissolve. Add the remaining salsa ingredients. Chill in the fridge for at least 30 minutes. Stir again just before using.

3. Lightly brush oil on both sides of tortillas. Cut these into large triangles.

4. Place a generous handful of sliced tortillas in the basket. Fry these for 10 minutes or until bread blisters and turns golden brown. Shake contents of the basket once midway through.

5. Place cooked pieces on a plate. Repeat step for remaining tortillas. Season with salt.

6. Place equal portions of crispy tortillas on plates. Serve with green mango and tomato salsa on the side.

Nutrition:

- Calories: 128
- Carbs: 8.6 g
- Fat: 3.6 g
- Protein: 2.7 g
- Fiber: 5.7 g

199.   Skinny Pumpkin Chips

Preparation Time: 20 minutes

Cooking Time: 13 minutes

Servings: 2

Ingredients:

- 1 lb. pumpkin, cut into sticks

- 1 tbsp. coconut oil
- 1/2 tsp. rosemary
- 1/2 tsp. basil
- Salt and ground black pepper to taste

Directions:

1. Start by preheating the air fryer to 395ºF. Brush the pumpkin sticks with coconut oil; add the spices and toss to combine.

2. Cook for 13 minutes, shaking the basket halfway through the cooking time.

3. Serve with mayonnaise. Enjoy!

Nutrition:

- Calories: 118
- Fat; 14.7 g
- Carbs; 2.2 g
- Protein; 6.2 g
- Sugars: 7 g

200.   Air Fried Ripe Plantains

Preparation Time: 10 minutes

Cooking Time: 10 minutes

Servings: 2

Ingredients:

- 2 pcs. large ripe plantain, peeled, sliced into inch thick disks
- 1 tbsp. coconut butter, unsweetened

Directions:

1. Preheat the air fryer to 350°F.
2. Brush a small amount of coconut butter on all sides of plantain disks.
3. Place one even layer into the air fryer basket, making sure none overlap or touch. Fry plantains for 10 minutes.
4. Remove from the basket. Place on plates. Repeat step for all plantains.
5. While plantains are still warm. Serve.

Nutrition:

- Calories: 209
- Carbs: 29 g
- Fat: 8 g
- Protein: 2.9 g
- Fiber: 3.5 g

201. Garlic Bread with Cheese Dip

Preparation Time: 10 minutes

Cooking Time: 5 minutes

Servings: 4

Ingredients:

- Fried garlic bread
- 1 medium baguette, halved lengthwise, cut sides toasted
- 2 garlic cloves, whole
- 4 tbsp. extra-virgin olive oil
- 2 tbsp. fresh parsley, minced

Blue cheese dip:

- 1 tbsp. fresh parsley, minced
- 1/4 cup fresh chives, minced
- 1/4 tsp. Tabasco sauce
- 1 tbsp. lemon juice, freshly squeezed
- 1/2 cup Greek yogurt, low fat
- 1/4 cup blue cheese, reduced fat
- 1/16 tsp. salt
- 1/16 tsp. white pepper

Directions:

1. Preheat the machine to 400°F.
2. Mix oil and parsley in a small bowl.
3. Vigorously rub garlic cloves on cut/toasted sides of the baguette. Dispose of garlic nubs.
4. Using a pastry brush, spread parsley-infused oil on the cut side of the bread.
5. Place the bread cut-side down on a chopping board. Slice into inch-thick half-moons.
6. Place bread slices in an air fryer basket. Fry for 3 to 5 minutes or until bread browns a little. Shake contents of the basket once midway through. Place cooked pieces on a serving platter. Repeat the step for the remaining bread.
7. To prepare blue cheese dip, mix all the ingredients in a bowl.
8. Place equal portions of fried bread on plates. Serve with blue cheese dip on the side.

Nutrition:

- Calories: 209
- Carbs: 29 g
- Fat: 8 g
- Protein: 2.9 g
- Fiber: 3.5 g

202.   Fried Mixed Veggies with Avocado Dip

Preparation Time: 10 minutes

Cooking Time: 10 minutes

Servings: 4

Ingredients:

- Oil for spraying
- 1 cup panko breadcrumbs. Add more if needed
- 1 large egg, whisked, add more if needed
- 1 cup all-purpose flour, add more if needed
- 1/8 tsp. flaky sea salt

Avocado-feta dip:

- 1 avocado, pitted, peeled, flesh scooped out
- 4 oz. feta cheese, reduced fat
- 2 leeks, minced
- 1 lime, freshly squeezed
- 1/4 cup fresh parsley, chopped roughly
- 1/16 tsp. black pepper
- 1/16 tsp. salt

Vegetables:

- 1 zucchini, sliced into matchsticks
- 1 carrot, sliced into matchsticks
- 1 parsnip, sliced into matchsticks

Directions:

1. Preheat the air fryer to 400°F.
2. Season carrots, parsnips, and zucchini with salt.
3. Dredge carrots with flour first, then dip them into the whisked egg, and finally into breadcrumbs. Place breaded pieces on a baking sheet lined with parchment paper. Repeat the step for all carrots. Then do the same for parsnips and zucchini.
4. Lightly spray vegetables with oil. Place a generous handful of carrots in the air fryer basket. Fry for 10 minutes or until breading turns golden brown, shaking contents of the basket once midway. Place cooked pieces on a plate. Repeat the step for the remaining carrots.
5. Do the preceding step for parsnips and then zucchini.
6. For the dip, except for salt, place the remaining ingredients in a food processor. Pulse a couple of times, and then process to desired consistency scraping down sides of the machine often. Taste. Add salt only if needed. Place in an airtight container. Chill until needed.

7. Place equal portions of cooked vegetables on plates. Serve with a small amount of avocado-feta dip on the side.

Nutrition:

- Calories: 109
- Carbs: 4.0 g
- Fat: 2.6 g
- Protein: 2.9 g
- Fiber: 2.5 g

203. Air Fried Plantains in Coconut Sauce

Preparation Time: 10 minutes

Cooking Time: 10 minutes

Servings: 4

Ingredients:

- 6 ripe plantains, peeled, quartered lengthwise
- 1 can coconut cream
- 2 tbsp. of honey
- 1 tbsp. of coconut oil

Directions:

1. Preheat the air fryer to 330°F.
2. Pour coconut cream in a thick-bottomed saucepan set over high heat; bring to boil. Reduce heat to lowest setting; simmer uncovered until the cream is reduced by half and darkens in color. Turn off heat.

3. Whisk in honey until smooth. Cool completely before using. Lightly grease a non-stick skillet with coconut oil.
4. Layer plantains in the air fryer basket and fry for 10 minutes or until golden on both sides; drain on paper towels. Place plantain on plates.
5. Drizzle in a small amount of coconut sauce. Serve.

Nutrition:

- Calories: 236
- Carbs: 0 g
- Fat: 1.5 g
- Protein: 1 g
- Fiber: 1.8 g

204. Beef and Mango Skewers

Preparation Time: 10 minutes

Cooking Time: 4−7 minutes

Servings: 4

Ingredients:

- 3/4 lb. (340 g) of beef sirloin tip, cut into 1-inch cubes
- 2 tbsp. balsamic vinegar
- 1 tbsp. olive oil
- 1 tbsp. honey
- 1/2 tsp. dried marjoram
- Pinch salt

- Freshly ground black pepper to taste
- 1 mango

Directions:

1. Put the beef cubes in a medium bowl and add the balsamic vinegar, olive oil, honey, marjoram, salt, and pepper. Mix well, then rub the marinade into the beef with your hands. Set aside.
2. To prepare the mango, stand it on end and cut the skin off using a sharp knife. Then carefully cut around the oval pit to remove the flesh. Cut the mango into 1-inch cubes.
3. Thread metal skewers alternating with 3 beef cubes and 2 mango cubes. Place the skewers in the air fryer basket.
4. Air fry at 390°F (199°C) for 4 to 7 minutes or until the beef is browned and at least 145°F (63°C).

Nutrition:

- Calories: 245
- Fat: 9 g
- Protein: 26 g
- Carbs: 15 g
- Fiber: 1 g
- Sugar: 14 g
- Sodium: 96 mg

205.   Kale Chips with Lemon Yogurt Sauce

Preparation Time: 10 minutes

Cooking Time: 5 minutes

Servings: 4

Ingredients:

- 1 cup plain Greek yogurt
- 3 tbsp. freshly squeezed lemon juice
- 2 tbsp. honey mustard
- 1/2 tsp. dried oregano
- 1 bunch curly kale
- 2 tbsp. olive oil
- 1/2 tsp. salt
- 1/8 tsp. pepper

Directions:

1. In a small bowl, mix the yogurt, lemon juice, honey mustard, and oregano, and set aside.
2. Remove the stems and ribs from the kale with a sharp knife. Cut the leaves into 2 to 3-inch pieces.
3. Toss the kale with olive oil, salt, and pepper. Rub the oil into the leaves with your hands.
4. Air fry the kale in batches at 390°F (199°C) until crisp, about 5 minutes, shaking the basket once during cooking time. Serve with the yogurt sauce.

Nutrition:

- Calories: 155
- Fat: 8 g
- Protein: 8 g
- Carbs: 13 g
- Fiber: 1 g
- Sugar: 3 g
- Sodium: 378 mg

206. Basil Pesto Bruschetta

Preparation Time: 10 minutes

Cooking Time: 4–8 minutes

Servings: 4

Ingredients:

- 8 slices French bread, ½-inch thick
- 2 tbsp. softened butter
- 1 cup shredded Mozzarella cheese
- 1/2 cup basil pesto
- 1 cup chopped grape tomatoes
- 2 green onions, thinly sliced

Directions:

1. Spread the bread with the butter and place butter-side up in the air fryer basket. Bake at 350ºF (177ºC) for 3 to 5 minutes or until the bread is light golden brown.
2. Remove the bread from the basket and top each piece with some of the cheese. Return

to the basket in batches and bake until the cheese melts for about 1 to 3 minutes.

3. Meanwhile, combine the pesto, tomatoes, and green onions in a small bowl.
4. When the cheese has melted, remove the bread from the air fryer and place it on a serving plate. Top each slice with some of the pesto mixture and serve.

Nutrition:

- Calories: 463
- Fat: 25 g
- Protein: 19 g
- Carbs: 41 g
- Fiber: 3 g
- Sugar: 2 g
- Sodium: 822 mg

207. Cinnamon Pear Chips

Preparation Time: 15 minutes

Cooking Time: 9–13 minutes

Servings: 4

Ingredients:

- 2 firm Bosc pears, cut crosswise into 1/8-inch-thick slices
- 1 tbsp. freshly squeezed lemon juice
- 1/2 tsp. ground cinnamon
- 1/8 tsp. ground cardamom or ground nutmeg

Directions:

1. Separate the smaller stem-end pear rounds from the larger rounds with seeds. Remove the core and seeds from the larger slices. Sprinkle all slices with lemon juice, cinnamon, and cardamom.

2. Put the smaller chips into the basket. Air fry at 380°F (193°C) for 3 to 5 minutes, until light golden brown, shaking the basket once during cooking. Remove from the air fryer.

3. Repeat with the larger slices, air frying for 6 to 8 minutes, until light golden brown, shaking the basket once during cooking.

4. Remove the chips from the air fryer. Cool and serve or store in an airtight container at room temperature for up to 2 days.

Nutrition:

- Calories: 31
- Fat: 0 g
- Protein: 7 g
- Carbs: 8 g
- Fiber: 2 g
- Sugar: 5 g
- Sodium: 0 mg

208. Phyllo Vegetable Triangles

Preparation Time: 15 minutes

Cooking Time: 6–11 minutes

Servings: 2

Ingredients:

- 3 tbsp. minced onion
- 2 garlic cloves, minced
- 2 tbsp. grated carrot
- 1 tsp. olive oil
- 3 tbsp. frozen baby peas, thawed
- 2 tbsp. non-fat cream cheese, at room temperature
- 6 sheets frozen phyllo dough, thawed
- Olive oil spray for coating the dough

Directions:

1. In a baking pan, combine the onion, garlic, carrot, and olive oil. Air fry at 390°F (199°C) for 2 to 4 minutes, or until the vegetables are crisp-tender. Transfer to a bowl.

2. Stir in the peas and cream cheese to the vegetable mixture. Let it cool while you prepare the dough.

3. Lay one sheet of phyllo on a work surface and lightly spray with olive oil spray. Top with another sheet of phyllo. Repeat with the remaining 4 phyllo sheets; you'll have 3 stacks with 2 layers each. Cut each stack lengthwise into 4 strips (12 strips total).

4. Place a scant 2 tsp. of the filling near the bottom of each strip. Bring one corner up over the filling to make a triangle; continue folding the triangles over, as you would fold

a flag. Seal the edge with a bit of water. Repeat with the remaining strips and filling.

5. Air fry the triangles, in 2 batches, for 4 to 7 minutes or until golden brown. Serve.

Nutrition:

- Calories: 67
- Fat: 2 g
- Protein: 2 g
- Carbs: 11 g
- Fiber: 1 g
- Sugar: 1 g
- Sodium: 121 mg

209.   Sweet Tapioca Pudding

Preparation Time: 10 minutes

Cooking Time: 8 minutes

Servings: 4

Ingredients:

- 1/2 cup pearl tapioca
- 1 can coconut milk
- 1/2 cup water
- 4 tbsp. maple syrup
- 1 cup almond milk
- Pinch cardamom

Directions:

1. Soak tapioca in almond milk for 1 hour.

2. Combine all ingredients except water into the heat-safe bowl and cover the bowl with foil.

3. Pour 1/2 cup water into the air fryer oven, then place trivet into the pot.

4. Place bowl on top of the trivet.

5. Cover pot with lid and cook on manual high pressure for 8 minutes.

6. Once done, allow to release pressure naturally, then open the lid.

7. Stir well—place in the refrigerator for 1 hour.

8. Serve and enjoy.

Nutrition:

- Calories: 313
- Fat: 18.1 g
- Carbs: 38.4 g
- Sugar: 18.5 g
- Protein: 2.4 g
- Cholesterol: 1 mg

210.   Vanilla Bread Pudding

Preparation Time: 10 minutes

Cooking Time: 15 minutes

Servings: 4

Ingredients:

- 3 eggs, lightly beaten
- 1 tsp. coconut oil
- 1 tsp. vanilla
- 4 cups bread cube
- 1/2 tsp. cinnamon

- 1/4 cup raisins
- 1/4 cup chocolate chips
- 2 cups milk
- 1/4 tsp. salt
- 2 cups of water

Directions:

1. Empty water into the air fryer oven then place trivet into the pot.
2. Add bread cubes to the baking dish.
3. In a large bowl, mix the remaining ingredients.
4. Pour bowl mixture into the baking dish on top of bread cubes and cover the dish with foil.
5. Abode the baking dish on top of the trivet.
6. Seal pot with lid and cook on steam mode for 15 minutes.
7. Once done, allow to release pressure naturally, then open the lid.
8. Carefully remove the baking dish from the pot.
9. Serve and enjoy.

Nutrition:

- Calories: 230
- Fat: 10.1 g
- Carbs: 25 g
- Sugar: 16.7 g
- Protein: 9.2 g
- Cholesterol: 135 mg

132. Blueberry Cupcakes

Preparation Time: 10 minutes

Cooking Time: 25 minutes

Servings: 4

Ingredients:

- 2 eggs, lightly beaten
- 1/4 cup butter, softened
- 1/2 tsp. baking soda
- 1 tsp. baking powder
- 1 tsp. vanilla extract
- 1/2 fresh lemon juice
- 1 lemon zest
- 1/4 cup sour cream
- 1/4 cup milk
- 1 cup sugar
- 3/4 cup fresh blueberries
- 1 cup all-purpose flour
- 1/4 tsp. salt
- 1 cup water

Directions:

1. Swell all ingredients into the large bowl and mix well.
2. Empty 1 cup water into the air fryer oven, then place trivet into the pot.
3. Pour batter into the silicone cupcake mound and place on top of the trivet.

4. Seal pot with lid and cook manual high pressure for 25 minutes.

5. Once done, allow to release pressure naturally, then open the lid.

6. Serve and enjoy.

Nutrition:

- Calories: 330
- Fat: 11.6 g
- Carbs: 53.6 g
- Sugar: 36 g
- Protein: 4.9 g
- Cholesterol: 80 mg

133. Moist Pumpkin Brownie

Preparation Time: 10 minutes

Cooking Time: 35 minutes

Servings: 4

Ingredients:

- 2 eggs, lightly beaten
- 3/4 cup pumpkin puree
- 1/2 tsp. baking powder
- 1/3 cup cocoa powder
- 1/2 cup almond flour
- 1 tbsp. vanilla
- 1/4 cup milk
- 1 cup maple syrup
- 2 cups water

- Cooking spray

Directions:

1. Swell all ingredients into the large bowl, and mix until well combined.

2. Spray spring-form pan with cooking spray.

3. Pour batter into the pan and cover it with foil.

4. Pour 2 cups of water into the air fryer oven and place trivet into the pot.

5. Abode the cake pan on top of the trivet.

6. Closure pot with lid and cook on manual mode for 35 minutes.

7. Once done, release pressure using the quick-release method, then open the lid.

8. Slice and serve.

Nutrition:

- Calories: 306
- Fat: 5.5 g
- Carbs: 62.9 g
- Sugar: 49.9 g
- Protein: 5.8 g
- Cholesterol: 83 mg

134. Mini Choco Cake

Preparation Time: 10 minutes

Cooking Time: 9 minutes

Servings: 2

Ingredients:

- 2 eggs

- 2 tbsp. swerve
- 1/4 cup cocoa powder
- 1/2 tsp. vanilla
- 1/2 tsp. baking powder
- 2 tbsp. heavy cream
- 1 cup water
- Cooking spray

Directions:

1. In a container, blend all dry ingredients until combined.
2. Swell all wet ingredients to the dry mixture and whisk until smooth.
3. Spray 2 ramekins with cooking spray.
4. Empty 1 cup water into the air fryer oven, then place trivet to the pot.
5. Pour batter into the ramekins and place ramekins on top of the trivet.
6. Closure pot with lid and cook on manual high pressure for 9 minutes.
7. Once done, release pressure using the quick-release method, then open the lid.
8. Carefully remove ramekins from the pot and let it cool.
9. Serve and enjoy.

Nutrition:

- Calories: 143
- Fat: 11.3 g
- Carbs: 15.7 g
- Protein: 7.8 g

- Cholesterol: 184 mg

135.   Cinnamon Pears

Preparation Time: 10 minutes

Cooking Time: 7 minutes

Servings: 4

Ingredients:

- 4 firm pears, peel
- 1/2 tsp. nutmeg
- 1/3 cup sugar
- 1 tsp. ginger
- 1 ½ tsp. cinnamon cloves
- 1 cinnamon stick
- 1 cup orange juice

Directions:

1. Add orange juice and all spices into the air fryer oven.
2. Place trivet into the pot.
3. Arrange pears on top of the trivet.
4. Closure pot with lid and cook on manual high pressure for 7 minutes.
5. Once done, allow to release pressure naturally, then open the lid.
6. Carefully remove pears from the pot and set aside.
7. Discard cinnamon stick and cloves from the pot.

8. Add sugar to the pot and set the pot on "Sauté" mode.

9. Cook sauce until thickened.

10. Pour sauce over pears and serve.

Nutrition:

- Calories: 221
- Fat: 0.6 g
- Carbs: 57.5 g
- Sugar: 42.4 g
- Protein: 1.3 g
- Cholesterol: 0 mg

136. Delicious Pumpkin Pudding

Preparation Time: 10 minutes

Cooking Time: 20 minutes

Servings: 4

Ingredients:

- 2 large eggs, lightly beaten
- 1/2 cup milk
- 1/2 tsp. vanilla
- 1 tsp. pumpkin pie spice
- 14 oz. pumpkin puree
- 3/4 cup swerve
- 1 ½ cup water
- Cooking spray

Directions:

1. Lard baking dish with cooking spray and set aside.

2. In a large bowl, whisk eggs with the remaining ingredients.

3. Empty 1 1/2 cup of water into the air fryer oven, then place a steamer rack in the pot.

4. Pour mixture into the prepared dish and cover with foil.

5. Place dish on top of steamer rack.

6. Closure pot with lid and cook on manual high pressure for 20 minutes.

7. As soon as done, discharge pressure naturally for 10 minutes and then release it using the quick-release method. Open the lid.

8. Carefully remove the dish from the pot and let it cool.

9. Place pudding dish in the refrigerator for 7 to 8 hours.

10. Serve and enjoy.

Nutrition:

- Calories: 58
- Fat: 2.3 g
- Carbs: 36.7 g
- Sugar: 33.3 g
- Protein: 3.5 g
- Cholesterol: 64 mg

137. Saffron Rice Pudding

Preparation Time: 10 minutes

Cooking Time: 12 minutes

Servings: 4

Ingredients:

- 1/2 cup rice
- 1/2 tsp. cardamom powder
- 3 tbsp. almonds, chopped
- 3 tbsp. walnuts, chopped
- 4 cups milk
- 1/2 cup sugar
- 2 tbsp. shredded coconut
- 1 tsp. saffron
- 3 tbsp. raisins
- 1 tbsp. ghee
- 1/8 tsp. salt
- 1/2 cup water

Directions:

1. Add ghee into the pot and set the pot on "Sauté" mode.
2. Add rice and cook for 30 seconds.
3. Add 3 cups milk, coconut, raisins, saffron, nuts, cardamom powder, sugar, 1/2 cup water, and salt and blending well.
4. Closure pot with lid and cook on manual high pressure for 10 minutes.
5. Once done, release pressure naturally for 15 minutes and then release it using the quick-release method. Open the lid.
6. Add remaining milk and stir well and cook on "Sauté" mode for 2 minutes.
7. Serve and enjoy.

Nutrition:

- Calories 280
- Fat: 9.9 g
- Carbs: 42.1 g
- Sugar: 27 g
- Protein: 8.2 g
- Cholesterol: 19 mg

138. Flavorful Carrot Halva

Preparation Time: 10 minutes

Cooking Time: 10 minutes

Servings: 4

Ingredients:

- 2 cups carrots, shredded
- 2 tbsp. ghee
- 1/2 tsp. cardamom
- 3 tbsp. ground cashews
- 1/4 cup sugar
- 1 cup milk
- 4 tbsp. raw cashews

- 3 tbsp. raisins

Directions:

1. Add ghee to the air fryer oven and set the pot on "Sauté" mode.
2. Add raisins and cashews and cook until lightly golden brown.
3. Add remaining ingredients except for cardamom and blending well.
4. Closure pot with lid and cook on manual high pressure for 10 minutes.
5. Once done, allow to release pressure naturally, then open the lid.
6. Add cardamom and stir well and serve.

Nutrition:

- Calories: 171
- Fat: 9.3 g
- Carbs: 20.5 g
- Sugar: 15.2 g
- Protein: 3.3 g
- Cholesterol: 14 mg

139. Vermicelli Pudding

Preparation Time: 10 minutes

Cooking Time: 2 minutes

Servings: 4

Ingredients:

- 1/3 cup vermicelli, roasted

- 6 dates, pitted, sliced
- 3 tbsp. cashews, slice
- 2 tbsp. pistachios, slice
- 1/4 tsp. vanilla
- 1/2 tsp. saffron
- 1/3 cup sugar
- 5 cups milk
- 3 tbsp. shredded coconut
- 2 tbsp. raisins
- 3 tbsp. almonds
- 2 tbsp. ghee

Directions:

1. Add ghee to the air fryer oven and set the pot on "Sauté" mode.
2. Add dates, cashews, pistachios, and almonds into the pot and cook for a minute.
3. Add raisins, coconut, and vermicelli. Stir well.
4. Add 3 cups of milk, saffron, and sugar. Blending well.
5. Closure pot with lid and cook on manual high pressure for 2 minutes.
6. Once done, allow to release pressure naturally, then open the lid.
7. Stir remaining milk and vanilla.
8. Serve and enjoy.

Nutrition:

- Calories: 283
- Fat: 13.4 g
- Carbs: 34.9 g

- Sugar: 28.1 g
- Protein: 9 g
- Cholesterol: 28 mg

140.   Yogurt Custard

Preparation Time: 10 minutes

Cooking Time: 20 minutes

Servings: 4

Ingredients:

- 1 cup plain yogurt
- 1 ½ tsp. ground cardamom
- 1 cup sweetened condensed milk
- 1 cup milk

Directions:

1. Add all ingredients into the heat-safe bowl and stir to combine.
2. Cover bowl with foil.
3. Pour 2 cups of water into the air fryer oven, then place the trivet in the pot.
4. Place bowl on top of the trivet.
5. Closure pot with lid and cook on manual high pressure for 20 minutes.
6. Once done, release pressure naturally for 20 minutes and then release it using the quick-release method. Open the lid.
7. Once the custard bowl is cool, then place it in the refrigerator for 1 hour.
8. Serve and enjoy.

Nutrition:

- Calories: 215
- Fat: 5.8 g
- Carbs: 33 g
- Sugar: 32.4 g
- Protein: 7.7 g
- Cholesterol: 23 mg

141.   Simple Raspberry Mug Cake

Preparation Time: 10 minutes

Cooking Time: 10 minutes

Servings: 3

Ingredients:

- 3 eggs
- 1 cup almond flour
- 1/2 tsp. vanilla
- 1 tbsp. swerve
- 2 tbsp. chocolate chips
- 1/2 cup raspberries
- 2 cups water
- Pinch salt

Directions:

1. Swell all ingredients into the large bowl, and mix until well combined.
2. Pour 2 cups of water into the air fryer oven, then place a trivet in the pot.

3. Pour batter into the heat-safe mugs. Cover with foil and place on top of the trivet.

4. Closure pot with lid and cook on manual high pressure for 10 minutes.

5. Once done, release pressure using the quick-release method, then open the lid.

6. Serve and enjoy.

Nutrition:

- Calories: 326
- Fat: 25.3 g
- Carbs: 20 g
- Sugar: 11.3 g
- Protein: 11.3 g
- Cholesterol: 165 mg

142.   Chocolate Mousse

Preparation Time: 10 minutes

Cooking Time: 6 minutes

Servings: 2

Ingredients:

- 4 egg yolks
- 1 ½ cup water
- 1/2 cup sugar
- 1 tsp. vanilla
- 1 cup heavy cream
- 1/2 cup cocoa powder
- 1/2 cup milk
- 1/4 tsp. sea salt

Directions:

1. Whisk egg yolks in a bowl until combined.

2. In a saucepan, add cocoa, water, and sugar and whisk over medium heat until sugar is melted.

3. Add milk and cream to the saucepan and whisk to combine. Do not boil.

4. Add vanilla and salt and stir well.

5. Empty 1 1/2 cup water into the air fryer oven, then place a trivet in the pot.

6. Pour mixture into the ramekins and place on top of the trivet.

7. Closure pot with lid and cook on manual mode for 6 minutes.

8. Once done, release pressure using the quick-release method, then open the lid.

9. Serve and enjoy.

Nutrition:

- Calories: 235
- Fat: 14.1 g
- Carbs: 27.2 g
- Sugar: 21.5 g
- Protein: 5 g
- Cholesterol: 203 mg

143.   Cardamom Zucchini Pudding

Preparation Time: 10 minutes

Cooking Time: 10 minutes

Servings: 4

Ingredients:

- 1 3/4 cup zucchini, shredded
- 5 oz. milk
- 1 tsp. cardamom powder
- 1/3 cup sugar

Directions:

1. Add all ingredients except cardamom into the air fryer oven and blending well.
2. Closure pot with lid and cook on manual high pressure for 10 minutes.
3. As soon as done, discharge pressure naturally for 10 minutes and then release it using the quick-release method. Open the lid.
4. Stir in cardamom and serve.

Nutrition:

- Calories: 138
- Fat: 5 g
- Carbs: 22.1 g
- Sugar: 19.4 g
- Protein: 3 g
- Cholesterol: 16 mg

144. Yummy Strawberry Cobbler

Preparation Time: 10 minutes

Cooking Time: 12 minutes

Servings: 3

Ingredients:

- 1 cup strawberries, sliced
- 1/2 tsp. vanilla
- 1/3 cup butter
- 1 cup milk
- 1 tsp. baking powder
- 1/2 cup granulated sugar
- 1 ¼ cup all-purpose flour
- 1 ½ cup water
- Cooking spray

Directions:

1. In a huge container, add all ingredients except strawberries and stir to combine.
2. Add sliced strawberries and fold well.
3. Grease ramekins with cooking spray, then pour batter into them.
4. Discharge 1 1/2 cup water into the air fryer oven, then place the trivet in the pot.
5. Place ramekins on top of the trivet.
6. Closure pot with lid and cook on manual high pressure for 12 minutes.
7. As soon as done, discharge pressure naturally for 10 minutes and then release it using the quick-release method. Open the lid.
8. Serve and enjoy.

Nutrition:

- Calories: 555
- Fat: 22.8 g
- Carbs: 81.7 g
- Sugar: 39.6 g
- Protein: 8.6 g
- Cholesterol: 61 mg

CHAPTER 17. FIRST 30-DAY MEAL PLAN

Day	Breakfast	Lunch	Dinner	Desserts/ Snacks
1	Coconut Pancakes	Tilapia With Coconut Rice	Oven-Baked Potatoes and Green Beans	Apple Crisp
2	Quinoa Porridge	Spicy Turkey Tacos	Hummus and Salad Pita Flats	Apple Pear and Pecan Dessert Squares
3	Amaranth Porridge	Quick and Easy Shrimp Stir-Fry	Lettuce Salad With Lemon	Apricot Soufflé
4	Overnight Oatmeal With Berries and Nuts	Chicken Burrito Bowl With Quinoa	Pork Chops and Butternut Squash Salad	Autumn Skillet Cake
5	Mushroom Breakfast Burrito	Baked Salmon Cakes	Low Carb Stuffed Peppers	Baked Maple Custard
6	No-Bake Blueberry Oats Bites	Rice and Meatball Stuffed Bell Peppers	Chicken Cordon Bleu	Blackberry Crostata
7	Avocado and Egg on Whole Wheat Toast	Stir-Fried Steak and Cabbage	Beef Goulash	Blackberry Soufflés
8	A Cup of Cottage Cheese With Peach Slices	Lemon Chicken With Peppers	Cajun Beef and Rice Skillet	Blueberry Lemon "Cup" Cakes
9	Peanut Butter Sandwich With Strawberry Jam	Dijon Herb Chicken	Cheesy Beef and Noodles	Blueberry No Bake Cheesecake
10	Chicken Nacho Casserole	Sesame Chicken Stir Fry	Bone Broth	Broiled Stone Fruit

11	Stir-Fried Vegetable and Egg Omelet	Rosemary Chicken	Tofu Mushrooms	Café Mocha Torte
12	Banana and Berry Smoothie	Pepper Chicken Skillet	Onion Tofu	Cappuccino Mousse
13	Make-Ahead Breakfast Quiche	Dijon Salmon	Spinach Rich Ballet	Caramel Pecan Pie
14	Cheesy Ham and Hash Casserole	Pulled Pork	Pepperoni Egg Omelet	Carrot Cupcakes
15	Egg and Bacon Tacos	Herb Lemon Salmon	Nut Porridge	Chocolate Cherry Cake Roll
16	Breakfast Crepes	Ginger Chicken	Parsley Soufflé	Chocolate Orange Bread Pudding
17	No-Bake Nut Butter Protein Bites	Teriyaki Chicken	Eggs and Ham	Chocolate Torte
18	Chicken on Whole Wheat Toast With Olive Oil	Roasted Garlic Salmon	Spicy Keto Chicken Wings	Cinnamon Bread Pudding
19	Egg and Avocado Omelet	Lemon Sesame Halibut	Sesame-Crusted Tuna With Green Beans	Coconut Cream Pie
20	Apple and Cinnamon Overnight Oats	Turkey Sausage Casserole	Grilled Salmon and Zucchini With Mango Sauce	Coconut Milk Shakes
21	Egg Muffin	Spinach Curry	Slow-Cooker Pot Roast With Green Beans	Cheesy Pita Crisps

22	Blueberry and Nuts Overnight Oats	Tilapia With Coconut Rice	Oven-Baked Potatoes and Green Beans	Cheesy Taco Chips
23	Apple and Cinnamon Pancakes	Spicy Turkey Tacos	Hummus and Salad Pita Flats	Chewy Granola Bars
24	Apple Pancakes	Quick and Easy Shrimp Stir-Fry	Lettuce Salad With Lemon	Chili Lime Tortilla Chips
25	Coconut Pancakes	Chicken Burrito Bowl With Quinoa	Pork Chops and Butternut Squash Salad	Chocolate Chip Blondies
26	Quinoa Porridge	Baked Salmon Cakes	Low Carb Stuffed Peppers	Cinnamon Apple Chips
27	Amaranth Porridge	Rice and Meatball Stuffed Bell Peppers	Chicken Cordon Bleu	Coffee-Steamed Carrots
28	Overnight Oatmeal With Berries And Nuts	Stir-Fried Steak And Cabbage	Beef Goulash	Rosemary Potatoes
29	Mushroom Breakfast Burrito	Lemon Chicken With Peppers	Cajun Beef and Rice Skillet	Fantastic Butternut Squash and Vegetables
30	No-Bake Blueberry Oats Bites	Dijon Herb Chicken	Cheesy Beef and Noodles	Fabulous Glazed Carrots

CHAPTER 18. SECOND 30-DAY MEAL PLAN

Day	Breakfast	Lunch	Dinner	Desserts/Snacks
1	Country-Style Pork Ribs	Salmon Cakes in Air Fryer	Duo Crisp Chicken Wings	Sweet Tapioca Pudding
2	Lemon and Honey Pork Tenderloin	Coconut Shrimp	Italian Whole Chicken	Vanilla Bread Pudding
3	Dijon Pork Tenderloin	Crispy Fish Sticks in Air Fryer	Chicken Pot Pie	Blueberry Cupcakes
4	Pork Satay	Honey-Glazed Salmon	Chicken Casserole	Moist Pumpkin Brownie
5	Pork Burgers with Red Cabbage Slaw	Basil-Parmesan Crusted Salmon	Ranch Chicken Wings	Mini Choco Cake
6	Breaded Pork Chops	Cajun Shrimp in Air Fryer	Chicken Mac and Cheese	Cinnamon Pears
7	Pork Taquitos in Air Fryer	Crispy Air Fryer Fish	Broccoli Chicken Casserole	Delicious Pumpkin Pudding
8	Tasty Egg Rolls	Air Fryer Lemon Cod	Chicken Tikka Kebab	Saffron Rice Pudding

9	Pork Dumplings	Air Fryer Salmon Fillets	Bacon-Wrapped Chicken	Flavorful Carrot Halva
10	Pork Chop & Broccoli	Air Fryer Fish and Chips	Creamy Chicken Thighs	Vermicelli Pudding
11	Eggplant Surprise	Grilled Salmon with Lemon	Air Fryer Teriyaki Hen Drumsticks	Sweet Tapioca Pudding
12	Carrots and Turnips	Air-Fried Fish Nuggets	Duo Crisp Chicken Wings	Vanilla Bread Pudding
13	Instant Brussels Sprouts With Parmesan	Garlic Rosemary Grilled Prawns	Italian Whole Chicken	Blueberry Cupcakes
14	Braised Fennel	Salmon Cakes in Air Fryer	Chicken Pot Pie	Moist Pumpkin Brownie
15	Brussels Sprouts & Potatoes Dish	Coconut Shrimp	Chicken Casserole	Mini Choco Cake
16	Beet and Orange Salad	Greek Lamb Pita Pockets	Meatloaf Slider Wraps	Sweet Potato Fries
17	Endives Dish	Rosemary Lamb Chops	Double Cheeseburger	Cheese Sticks
18	Roasted Potatoes	Herb Butter Lamb Chops	Beef Schnitzel	Zucchini Crisps

19	Cabbage Wedges	Za'atar Lamb Chops	Steak with Asparagus Bundles	Tortillas in Green Mango Salsa
20	Creamed Spinach	Greek Lamb Chops	Hamburgers	Air Fried Ripe Plantains
21	Eggplant Parmesan	Herbed Lamb Chops	Beef Steak Kabobs with Vegetables	Garlic Bread with Cheese Dip
22	Eggplant Surprise	Spicy Lamb Sirloin Steak	Rib-Eye Steak	Fried Mixed Veggies with Avocado Dip
23	Carrots and Turnips	Garlic Rosemary Lamb Chops	Bunless Sloppy Joes	Air Fried Plantains in Coconut Sauce
24	Instant Brussels Sprouts With Parmesan	Cherry-Glazed Lamb Chops	Beef Curry	Beef and Mango Skewers
25	Braised Fennel	Lamb and Vegetable Stew	Asian Grilled Beef Salad	Kale Chips with Lemon Yogurt Sauce
26	Brussels Sprouts & Potatoes Dish	Lime-Parsley Lamb Cutlets	Sunday Pot Roast	Sweet Potato Fries
27	Beet and Orange Salad	Greek Lamb Pita Pockets	Beef Burrito Bowl	Cheese Sticks

28	Endives Dish	Rosemary Lamb Chops	Beef and Pepper Fajita Bowls	Zucchini Crisps
29	Roasted Potatoes	Herb Butter Lamb Chops	Meatloaf Slider Wraps	Tortillas in Green Mango Salsa
30	Cabbage Wedges	Za'atar Lamb Chops	Double Cheeseburger	Air Fried Ripe Plantains

CHAPTER 19. MEASUREMENT CONVERSION CHART

VOLUME EQUIVALENTS(DRY)

US STANDARD	METRIC (APPROXIMATE)
1/8 teaspoon	0.5 mL
1/4 teaspoon	1 mL
1/2 teaspoon	2 mL
3/4 teaspoon	4 mL
1 teaspoon	5 mL
1 tablespoon	15 mL
1/4 cup	59 mL
1/2 cup	118 mL
3/4 cup	177 mL
1 cup	235 mL
2 cups	475 mL
3 cups	700 mL
4 cups	1 L

VOLUME EQUIVALENTS(LIQUID)

US STANDARD	US STANDARD (OUNCES)	METRIC (APPROXIMATE)
2 tablespoons	1 fl.oz.	30 mL
1/4 cup	2 fl.oz.	60 mL
1/2 cup	4 fl.oz.	120 mL
1 cup	8 fl.oz.	240 mL
1 1/2 cup	12 fl.oz.	355 mL
2 cups or 1 pint	16 fl.oz.	475 mL
4 cups or 1 quart	32 fl.oz.	1 L
1 gallon	128 fl.oz.	4 L

TEMPERATURES EQUIVALENTS

FAHRENHEIT(F)	CELSIUS(C) (APPROXIMATE)
225 °F	107 °C
250 °F	120 °C
275 °F	135 °C
300 °F	150 °C
325 °F	160 °C
350 °F	180 °C
375 °F	190 °C
400 °F	205 °C
425 °F	220 °C
450 °F	235 °C
475 °F	245 °C
500 °F	260 °C

WEIGHT EQUIVALENTS

US STANDARD	METRIC (APPROXIMATE)
1 ounce	28 g
2 ounces	57 g
5 ounces	142 g
10 ounces	284 g
15 ounces	425 g
16 ounces (1 pound)	455 g
1.5 pounds	680 g
2 pounds	907 g

CONCLUSION

With the knowledge I have shared, you now know why you may have developed diabetes, you know what this means, and now, you also know how to manage it. You are armed with resources, apps, and recipes to help you along this lifelong journey. Food is not your enemy; it's your friend.

Cook your way to vitality and health with these recipes and tips. Good things are made for sharing, so please help a friend find out about this way of life. Call them over for a meal, talk about diabetes, and let's help create awareness as we feast on every delectable spoonful of diabetic cooking made easy.

The warning symptoms of diabetes type 1 are the same as type 2. However, in type 1, these signs and symptoms tend to occur slowly over months or years, making it harder to spot and recognize. Some of these symptoms can even occur after the disease has progressed.

Each disorder has risk factors that, when found in an individual, favor the development of the disease. Diabetes is no different.

Usually, having a family member, especially first-degree relatives, could indicate that you are at risk of developing diabetes. Your risk of diabetes is about 15% if you have one parent with diabetes, while it is 75% if both your parents have diabetes.

Being pre-diabetic means that you have higher than normal blood glucose levels. However, they are not high enough to be diagnosed as type 2 diabetes. Having pre-diabetes is a risk factor for developing type 2 diabetes as well as other conditions such as cardiac conditions. Since there are no symptoms or signs of pre-diabetes, it is often a latent condition that is discovered accidentally during routine investigations of blood glucose levels or when investigating other conditions.

Your metabolism, fat stores, and eating habits when you are overweight or above the healthy weight range contribute to abnormal metabolism pathways that put you at risk for developing diabetes type 2. There have been consistent research results of the obvious link between developing diabetes and being obese.

Having a lifestyle where you are most physically inactive predisposes you to a lot of conditions, including diabetes type 2. That is because being physically inactive causes you to develop obesity or become overweight.

Moreover, you don't burn any excess sugars that you ingest, which can lead you to become prediabetic and eventually diabetic.

Developing gestational diabetes, which is diabetes that occurred due to pregnancy (and often disappears after pregnancy) is a risk factor for developing diabetes at some point.

Belonging to certain ethnic groups such as Middle Eastern, South Asian, or Indian background. Studies of statistics have revealed that the prevalence of diabetes type 2 in these ethnic groups is high. If you come from any of these ethnicities, this puts you at risk of developing diabetes type 2 yourself.

Studies have shown an association between having hypertension and having an increased risk of developing diabetes. If you have hypertension, you should not leave it uncontrolled.

Diabetes can occur at any age. However, being too young or too old means your body is not in its best form, and therefore, this increases the risk of developing diabetes.

When your body is low on sugars, it will be forced to use a subsequent molecule to burn for energy. In that case, this will be fat. The burning of fat will lead you to lose weight.

I hope you have learned something!